MW01591072

I Love You Madly!
Workbook
Insight Enhancement about Healthy and Disturbed Love Relations

Robert M. Gordon, Ph.D.

The drawing on the cover is Cupid and Psyche by the 18th century artist Giuseppe Cammarano. Here Psyche is using her lamp to see the true nature of her mysterious night lover Cupid.

From my book, *I Love You Madly! On Passion, Personality, and Personal Growth.*

Alla had studied art and was, as she promised, my guide through the Hermitage Art Museum . . . "Apuleius tells this story in *Metamorphoses.* It is a story about us, my Swan! Here Eros—the Romans later called him Cupid—sees Psyche and falls in love with her. That angers Venus, his mother. So then Eros makes love to Psyche secretly in the dark. O-la la! When Psyche lit a lamp to see who he was, he awakens and flees. You see, Robert, some things like love are better left to mystery."

I said, "Eros could not stay with Psyche because he was too tied to his mother. So he could only play with passion and not commit. Only because of Psyche's courage do they marry. Psyche is the mother of my science. Psychology is a science that looks at passion so it might stay."

I Love You Madly! Workbook

Insight Enhancement about Healthy and Disturbed Love Relations

Robert M. Gordon, Ph.D.

ISBN 978-0-9779616-1-0

Library of Congress Control Number: 2007920832

New Yorker cartoons licensed through Cartoonbank.com.

First Printing 2007. IAPT Press, 1259 S. Cedar Crest Blvd., Suite 325, Allentown, Pa. 18103 For extra copies: Call AtlasBooks 1-800-247-6553 anytime 24/7 or go to www.bookmasters.com/marketplc/01825.htm, or www.mmpi-info.com.

Much of this workbook is based on my books, *I Love You Madly! On Passion, Personality and Personal Growth,* and *An Expert Look at Love, Intimacy and Personal Growth,* which can also be purchased at www.mmpi-info.com.

I dedicate this workbook to my loving wife and colleague Alla Gordon and to all my patients who deepened my understanding of the human condition.

Table of Contents

1. How this Workbook Works   1

2. What Is Love?   11

3. The Causes of Love and Its Disturbances   17

4. The Influence of Parenting on Later
   Love Relations   35

5. What Is Romantic Love?   63

6. What Are the Stages of Romantic Love?   67

7. What Are Disturbed Love Relations?   71

8. How Temperaments Affect Love Relations   79

9. How Defensive Styles Affect Love Relations   89

10. On Being Constructive   95

    References   101

How this Workbook Works

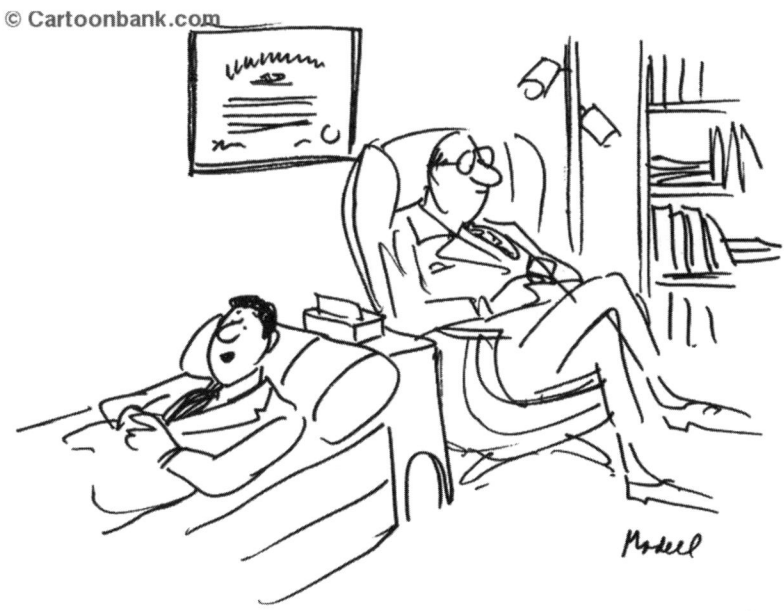

"And then I say to myself, 'If I really wanted to talk to her, why do I keep forgetting to dial 1 first?'"

How can this workbook help you?

This workbook can help you improve your insight so that you might have better love relations.

How is this workbook different from the others? It is based on time-tested treatment and the latest theoretical and scientific findings. It goes deeper than most.

What can you get from this book?

First, it can give you psychological information about the nature of intimacy.

Second, it can help you to apply this psychological information to yourself and your relationships.

Third, it will give you exercises to help you increase your insight.

The goal of these exercises is to increase your insight about love relations and love disturbances.

How can insight help?

What is insight? Insight involves a deep understanding of the reasons behind human behavior. Insight gives you the power to discern the true nature of yourself and others.

Some motives are conscious. Here is an example of a conscious motive. Sally sees that she is low on gasoline, so she consciously decides to get some. She decides what station to go to and how to get the gasoline into her car. She does so with no problems.

Emotional motives are usually unconsciously determined. When it comes to love relations, our motives are frequently unconscious and irrational.

For example, Sally was feeling low on love. She consciously decides to ask for some love from her partner. However, she complains and demands to such an extent that her partner rejects her. That is an example of an unconscious conflict expressing itself as a self-defeating motive.

Had Sally used insight, things might have turned out differently. She might have thought, "Why am I so angry, as if I have been cheated? He loves me. Where are these feelings coming from? I remember that as a child, my mother was depressed and had little emotional resources left for me. I felt unloved. If I expressed my anger at her, I might have hurt her. In addition, I might have pushed her away. That is not the case now.[1]"

---

[1]You might wonder if psychologists analyze all the time. We do not. However, it is nice to know that we can use insight when we need it.

Sally used insight to examine her motives. She remembered her past. By doing so, she distinguished it from the present. After using insight she said, "Honey, I am feeling low. I could use some loving." She was successful. She was not only successful for the moment in having her needs met, but she was, more importantly, on her way to personal growth. The more she applies insight, the less her conflicts from the past will harm her present.

With insight, your motives can be more conscious and more self-actualizing. I do not expect someone to constantly use insight as Sally did in our example. What I am suggesting is that it is hard to resolve problems if you have no understanding of the problem.

Personal growth depends on insight. However, defensiveness is the enemy of insight. You cannot have much personal growth or learn to love better if you are defensive. If you would rather prove that you are right than learn from your mistakes, you might as well not waste your time on this.

It is normal to want to have feedback that you are right, that you are fine just the way you are. Most everyone wants validation. Validation feels good, but it does not lead to change for the better. This workbook will be useless if it does not give you insights into areas where you can improve and have more satisfying intimacies.

If you are open to insight, you are on your way to personal growth.

How important is insight? Well, when 800 psychologists were surveyed about what THEY wanted from their OWN psychotherapy, do you know what was most important to them?

Psychologists ranked a list of 38 of the most beneficial things they got from their own psychotherapy. They listed first, "Self-understanding" (insight about one's self). The results of the survey had "symptom relief" as halfway down the list of 38 benefits. Included in the survey were psychologists from all theoretical orientations (Behaviorists, Cognitive-Behaviorists, Psychoanalytic, etc.) (Pope, 1994).

What psychologists understand is that symptom reduction without understanding the underlying problems is often not enough.[2]

---

[2]Behavioral and Cognitive Behavioral psychologists tend to seek insight therapy for themselves. However, many of these psychologists have to help patients who want relief from their symptoms and do not desire insight or personal growth.

Psychologists understand that insight into one's problems can lead to something deeper. Insight can lead to becoming a more effective problem solver in life. Psychologists do not look for stock answers for themselves. They work to become more perceptive, understanding, and mature. All this starts with insight.

How can this workbook help you with insight so you can have better intimacy? It is difficult to get personal growth without some form of insight psychotherapy. I cannot expect you to be honest if I am not. I have to be honest about the limitations of reading books. A book does not know your unique history and character. A book cannot challenge your blind spots. A book cannot develop a therapeutic relationship with you so you will have a safe place to explore deeper parts of your personality. A book will not tell you when you are wrong.

Real personal growth occurs in the context of a therapeutic intimacy (Norcross, 2002; Wampold, 2001). In the therapeutic intimacy found in insight psychotherapy, the patient unconsciously behaves towards the therapist in ways the patient does not see, nor can report. When the patient expresses the unconscious conflicts and defenses, the therapist can use insight in the context of the caring relationship.

This book works best in conjunction with a therapeutic relationship.

If you are currently in psychotherapy, this workbook might help you get over some blocks. It might help you to work deeper in psychotherapy. On the other hand, if you had been in psychotherapy, it might help you to continue some of your personal growth.

If you are not in a psychotherapeutic relationship, this workbook might help you to decide to go to psychotherapy and to do deeper self-improvement. Psychotherapy is the highest level of education, since its aim is to help you be a better person.

What is insight psychotherapy?

Therapists who are afraid to go into their own past and unconscious might claim that they do not believe that insight is important. This is fine if you need supportive therapy or symptom reduction therapy. However, if you want personal growth so that you can have more satisfying and meaningful intimacy, then you want a therapist who uses insights about intimacy. Insight psychotherapy deals with your self-defeating unconscious patterns that come from the interpersonal past and your personality traits.

Psychoanalysis is the deepest form of insight psychotherapy. It produces the most personal growth with those patients who have high abstract reasoning, insight, and a capacity for concern. To become a psychoanalyst requires about four to six years of intensive post doctorate training, supervision, and a personal/training psychoanalysis. It takes high intelligence, symbolic reasoning, and emotional maturity.

Sigmund Freud felt that psychoanalysis was one of the most important parts of a psychoanalyst's education. Freud wrote, "Every analyst ought periodically . . . to enter analysis once more, at intervals of, say, five years, and without any feeling of shame in doing so" (1937/1963).

Many patients who cannot afford the time and money for a full psychoanalysis may achieve a great deal of personal growth in psychoanalytic psychotherapy. Psychoanalytic psychotherapy is psychoanalysis, but with once or twice weekly sessions instead of the three to five sessions that are required for psychoanalysis.

Psychodynamic psychotherapy is a popular form of insight psychotherapy since it relies on insight, but it is often balanced between support, practical advice, and analysis of the unconscious.

Although Cognitive Behavior Therapy is not insight psychotherapy, it can help with some dysfunctional symptoms in relationships such as anger management, impulse problems, or communication skills. However, the insight psychotherapies (psychoanalysis, psychoanalytic psychotherapy, and psychodynamic psychotherapy) can go deeper to help people to love more maturely by focusing on transferences. Transferences are reactions to someone in the present because of a past relationship. Problems with love relations are often due to these unconscious transferences.

The problems with love relations are not in superficial habits or thoughts, but in unconscious deficits, conflicts, and defenses. It takes insight into these self-defeating unconscious patterns within

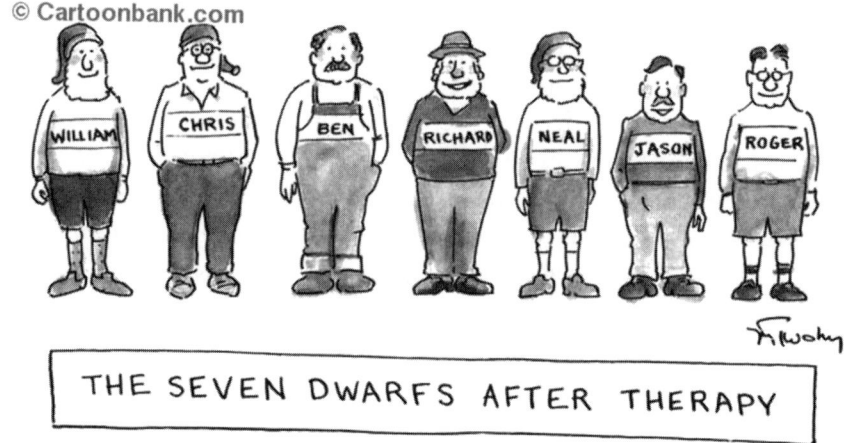

THE SEVEN DWARFS AFTER THERAPY

the context of a therapeutic intimacy to improve a person's love relations.

If you have unhappy love relations, the best thing you can do is to see a psychotherapist who will explore your unconscious self-defeating patterns. If you are already in psychotherapy, you might find these insight exercises helpful to your therapy.

Most of you might not be in psychotherapy. This book will ask you many of the same questions that I ask people in insight psychotherapy. I use these types of questions to help people create healthier relationships. These exercises might be all you need to begin your inspired personal growth.

If you find that these insights are a good start, but not enough, then you might want to go for insight psychotherapy.

Emotional versus intellectual insights

Self-help books have had a tremendous impact on society. They have reached millions of people and offered them helpful advice. Nevertheless, self-help books are of limited value. Even if you gain intellectual insights from reading, these insights remain isolated in the left (logical) part of the brain. These intellectual insights are isolated from the unconscious, more primitive part of the brain primarily associated with your emotions (Panksepp, 1998, 2004).

This workbook can at best provide you with insights for you to apply. I hope that you do the necessary work to move the intellectual insights to emotional insights and finally to constructive action. Intellectual insights do not necessarily affect emotional insights. Your emotional insights can affect the quality of your love relations. They can mediate the areas of the brain associated with the sex drive, attraction, and the attachment aspects of intimacy.

Emotional insights can lead to personal growth when you apply them in your intimacy. For example, an intellectual insight is that the relationship that you had with your parents as a child affects how you are intimate today.

You have an emotional insight when you emotionally connect the present problem in a relationship with a feeling and memory from childhood.

You need emotional insights to keep you from transferring past feelings onto current relationships. If you had a parent who had trouble understanding your feelings, your upset feelings would be stored in your unconscious (implicit) memory. Later in relationships, when your beloved does not understand you, this might be a trigger for old intense feelings.

Chronic empathic failures are dangerous to a child's self-esteem. A primary caregiver's lack of empathy damages a child. A primary caregiver damages the child without the child's conscious realization of this trauma. Later in adult intimacies, there are inevitable empathic failures. We are imperfect, and we all do annoying things. We do not always understand.

Our overreactions to misunderstandings can be a cue that there is probably a transference happening.

If you have an emotional insight, you will remember that empathic failures are a trigger based in childhood hurts and are not about anything dangerous now. Adults do not need empathy as children do. Children need empathy for healthy development. Adults value empathy for healthy intimacy. However, empathic failures are not dangerous—they are only disappointing. Putting this into perspective with emotional insight can change how you react to intimacy.

Research is clear that the parts of the brain that influence love relations are mainly unconscious (Buss, 1994; Fisher, 2000; Fonagy, 2002; Otto F. Kernberg, 1995). So how, then, do we know anything about something unconscious?

We can only deduce our unconscious issues by looking back at our life and seeing the patterns. It is hard for a book to interpret a person's unconscious patterns (however, I will try!).

Insight psychotherapy is the best place for exploring the unconscious, and psychoanalysis goes the deepest. I will give you an example from my book, *I Love You Madly! On Passion, Personality and Personal Growth* (Gordon, 2006b).

> My patient George had a hostile relationship with his alcoholic mother. He married young to escape her. He married an alcoholic woman. He divorced her and remarried. Alice, his second wife, was also an alcoholic.
>
> George protested when I suggested that he repeated his attachment with his mother in his love relations. George said, "Alice had stopped drinking before we first met. It was only after the second year of marriage that she began to drink again."
>
> George's urge to repeat his attachment pattern was unconscious. I interpreted, "You knew she once had a drinking problem and you could have unconsciously detected many of her personality traits that were similar to your mother's. Her traits triggered the feelings of idealization that you first had for your mother. This primitive idealization is the root of all love. That came long before you had any awareness of a conflict with your mother. When you fall in love, you would enact both sides of the emotions in your love relations, first idealization and then the old conflicts from childhood."
>
> George was not ready to concede that he had a goal-directed unconscious. "How is that possible? I saw her across the room at a party. It was love at first sight."
>
> I explained, "The human face has about thirty muscles that can be used for emotional expression. They can communicate many subtle messages. Our unconscious can read aspects of a person's personality and emotions from the face (Young, 1997). You were attracted to the way she looked, her nonverbal expressions, and then what she said. They were all triggers for your unconscious love drama."
>
> Over the many psychotherapy sessions, George began to see the patterns he was repeating in his relationships. Eventually he gained enough personal growth to love more wisely and develop passion for a much healthier woman.

George was only able to know about his unconscious patterns by reflecting on the interpretations. This workbook is asking you to do the same. First, read the information to begin to stimulate your intellectual insights. Then respond to the exercises to stimulate emotional insights. Remember, do not just think—*feel* what you are writing. It is a good idea to talk about these issues with someone insightful. Sometimes, hearing your voice as you talk about an issue can produce more insight. In addition, an honest dialogue can lead to deeper understanding.

Are there side effects?

There are no tests here. You cannot flunk. However, you may learn to better understand yourself and have intimacy that is more satisfying. Yet, many people do not learn from their mistakes. They may be too defensive and remain in their dysfunctional interpersonal patterns. This workbook is not for someone in denial. Do not use this workbook to prove to yourself or someone else that you are perfect.

Constructive feedback is crucial to personal growth. People with good self-esteem acknowledge their faults. You can increase your self-esteem by becoming more comfortable with all the sides of you.

Most people will not become distressed over these insight exercises. Most people might have feelings that motivate them to have useful insights. Some people may become upset when realizing how they contributed to their problems and/or how the past may hold some unfinished emotions.

If you experience too much distress, stop and try to self-sooth. Talk your feelings out with someone you trust. Ideally, that person will be a "good emotional container." He or she should not "validate" your defenses, nor give simplistic advice. That person only needs to listen and let you vent.

It is not a bad thing if this workbook stimulates some emotions that you wish to take to a psychotherapist or "therapeutic other." Learning more about yourself, and learning to be more loving are two of the most important things that you can do in life. You have already shown courage by reading these pages.

Remember the goals!

The goals of this book are to:

1. Learn about healthy versus disturbed love relations.
2. Increase your insight about yourself and others.
3. Learn how to have more satisfying love relations.

Do not rush through this workbook! Do not treat this as a pop-psych-fast-food drive through. Self-reflection takes time. Insight into deeper areas of your mind takes time. Personal growth takes lots of time. Learning to love well takes a lifetime.

I (Gordon, 2001) studied 55 polysymptomatic outpatients in psychoanalytic psychotherapy with objective testing (MMPI). After about three years of treatment, symptoms decreased by about 50 percent. There were major reductions in the areas of health complaints, depression, intimacy problems, anger, narcissism, anxiety, identity confusion, impulsiveness, and insecurity. However, not only were there reductions in symptoms, but there was also a significant increase in what psychoanalysts call "ego-strength." Ego-strength is a person's capacity for a realistic sense of self and others, objectivity, self-soothing and resiliency, healthy values, and judgment, which can affect tolerance and mature emotional expression. This sort of personal growth is possible with insight and hard work.

This workbook should take weeks to complete. Take a day on a section—or longer. Take the time to think, remember, and feel. I can work with a person for months in psychotherapy on just one of these issues. So go slow. Make it meaningful.

2
What Is Love?

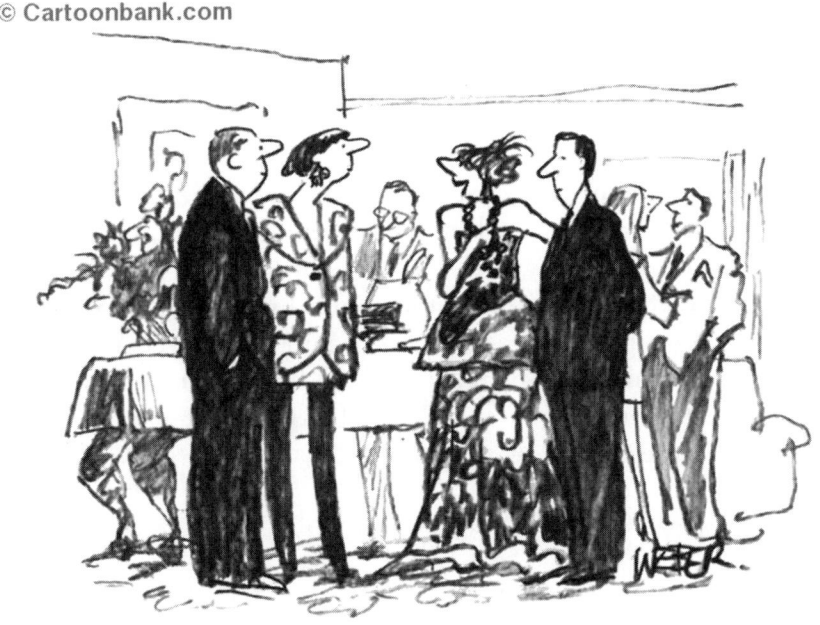

"Kevin's sort of a negative person, while I tend to be positive, so we have an electrical connection."

Sigmund Freud said that wherever he went in his study of love, he found that a poet was there before him. The artist can best convey love, but the scientist can better explain it. Does an analysis of love kill the appreciation of love? I do not think so. No more than studying art kills the appreciation of art. I believe that the more people understand themselves and the psychology of love, the better they can love. So then, what is love?

Freud (1912) believed that love required the balance of:

1. Passion
2. Tenderness

People seek passion in romantic love. Passion has components of sexuality and aggression. However, without tenderness, the aggressive aspect of passion may eventually consume and destroy the love relationship. Many relationships end because the aggression over time accumulates and wears down the love.

Some people with narcissistic personality traits can feel intense passion and have little sexual inhibitions. However, they have too much aggression and have difficulty in maintaining feelings of tenderness and concern.

There are those with neurotic traits (example: the main problems are with anxiety and/or depression) who can maintain feelings of tenderness and concern, but who struggle with guilt feelings and sexual inhibitions.

Too much narcissism or too much neurotic guilt will cause problems. One principle aim of psychoanalysis is to bring the passion and tenderness into a mature balance for healthy love relations.

Robert Sternberg, a social psychologist, (Sternberg, 1986a) theorized three components of love:

1. Intimacy
2. Passion
3. Commitment

Infatuation is based only on passion. Liking is based on intimacy. Romantic love has intimacy and passion. Companion love has intimacy and commitment without passion. Consummate love has all three—intimacy, passion, and commitment.

Helen Fisher (2000), an anthropologist, found that humans and other mammals have evolved three emotion systems in their brains that affect love relations:

1. Sex drive
2. Attraction
3. Attachment

Each emotion system is associated with a discrete constellation of brain circuits and each evolved to direct a specific aspect of mating, reproduction, and parenting.

Freud, Sternberg, and Fisher come from very different theoretical and research perspectives, but they agree that the success of love is dependent on all the parts working together. These parts include the ability to:

1. Commit
2. Maintain feelings of tenderness and concern for the other
3. Have passion without neurotic guilt

Generally, these parts do not come together well when people have a developmental arrest in their personalities because of early psychological trauma and/or temperamental disturbances.

Now, answer all these questions in the manner that best helps you understand yourself. Circle the number that comes closest to your HONEST opinion. If a question does not apply to you, write "NA."

How much passion do you feel in your current relationship?

None	Low		Medium		High
0	1	2	3	4	5

Why?

How much passion do you feel in your typical relationship?

None	Low		Medium		High
0	1	2	3	4	5

Why?

How much tenderness and concern do you express?

None	Low		Medium		High
0	1	2	3	4	5

Why?

How much commitment do you give?

None	Low		Medium		High
0	1	2	3	4	5

Why?

How much friendship do you express?

None	Low		Medium		High
0	1	2	3	4	5

Why?

How much love do you currently receive?

None	Low		Medium		High
0	1	2	3	4	5

Why?

How satisfied are you with your partner?

None	Low		Medium		High
0	1	2	3	4	5

Why?

What do these ratings tell you about your love relation(s)?

3
The Causes of Love and Its Disturbances

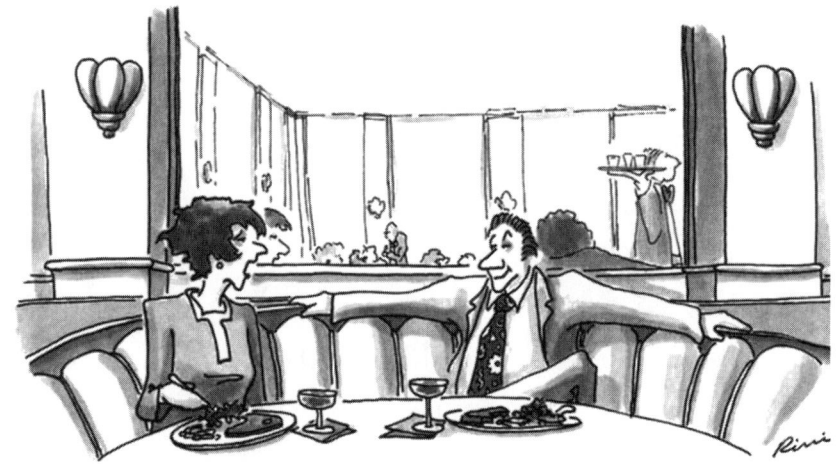

"Tell me, do you respond to treatment?"

I have developed a model to help understand why romantic love is so irrational (Gordon, 2006 d). It is a model that integrates the findings of evolutionary psychology, psychoanalysis, neuroscience, cognitive psychology, and social psychology. This workbook is unique in that it is founded in research and a new model of integrated psychology.

Imagine a pyramid that includes:

1. Who we are as humans
2. Who we are as an individual with an innate temperament
3. Our early attachment experiences

4. The effects of culture, learning, and beliefs
5. Current psychological context

Each level is a source of our motives and perceptions that affect how we love. (See figure 1.)

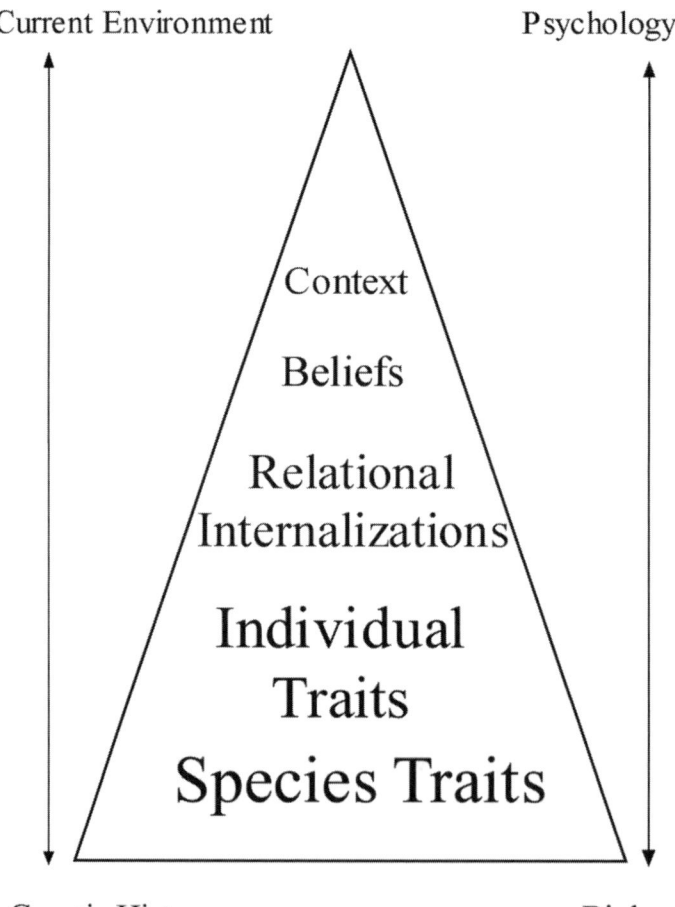

Current Environment   Psychology

Context

Beliefs

Relational
Internalizations

Individual
Traits

Species Traits

Genetic History   Biology

Figure 1: An Integrated Model of Factors Contributing to Love
          Relations

Species traits

At the base (primitive level) are our species traits that we possess as a result of natural selection. The instincts that affect our mating behaviors are 1. a sex drive, 2. triggers of attractiveness, and 3. an urge to bond (Fisher, 2000).

Our sex drive is innate from birth, but the development of sexuality is affected by all the levels. What we as humans tend to find attractive in a mate is partly based on what had survival value for our species. David Buss (1994) surveyed 10,047 people from 37 cultures. Buss reported that universally men preferred youthful, healthy-looking women, and women preferred men with attributes of success and power.

Buss believes that youthful, healthy-looking women provide triggers to their greater chance of bearing healthy offspring. Powerful and successful men are triggers for mating since they were both able to be protective of their mates and offspring and provide resources. In addition, attractive mates are able to pass on their valuable qualities to their children. These species traits remain with us regardless of our conscious interest in having children or sexual orientation. That is, these traits are common to all humans to some degree.

These are concrete and primitive triggers of passion. They create a temporary overidealization of a potential mate. They have worked in service to the evolution of our species. However, these instinctual triggers of passion have little to do with the success of love relations.

Mates need to experience at least a temporary sense of bonding to increase the odds of reproduction. In addition, bonding protects the offspring. This instinctive urge to bond in couples will naturally fade if it is not reinforced by an ongoing, rewarding love relationship.

As people mature, these instinctual motives become better integrated within their personality. Although passion is connected to the primitive side of the personality, with maturity, these primitive triggers to passion are contained within feelings of tenderness and concern for the other.

All love has some degree of idealization (overvaluing) of the beloved. However, the idealizations that come from our instinctual urges are the least likely to evolve into a lasting love. If your attraction is based mainly on these primitive instincts, it is not enough to last. For love to last there needs to also be a strong element of friendship, concern, and common values.

Individual traits

The next level involves individual traits, such as temperament. These traits are largely inborn and enduring.

Some traits are stressful for anyone, such as hostility. Some individual traits may clash with a partner's traits, such as when two people are both competitive. Other traits may complement each other; for example, a nurturing person and a dependent person may be compatible. Opposites tend to attract and have passion.

Although opposites attract, couples with similar goals and values get along better. Perhaps nature programmed opposites to mate. The diversity of personalities of parents may provide the offspring with a mix of genes and role models that have greater survival value. This may have worked in evolutionary history, but seems to work against a lasting marriage. Attraction is instinctual. Marriage is not. Its stability is dependent on the maturity and compatibility of the couple.

Couples seem to do best with some combination of differences that bring some complementarily and diversity of roles and some similarities in basic goals and values.

Emotional maturity is perhaps the most important factor in successful intimacy. Individuals with immature personality traits (example: borderline personality traits) tend to overidealize and then devalue the love object based on their own emotional fluctuations and primitive defenses (example: idealization/devaluation, splitting, and projection) (Kernberg, 1974, 1985, 1995, 2002). People who have personality traits such as over aggressiveness, egocentricity, and primitive defenses will have love disturbances with anyone. With primitive defense mechanisms, there are frequent distortions of a partner based on a person's internal problems. It is hard to have a normal relationship with a high degree of distortion of reality.

Individual traits can create an idealization of the love object based on projection. When attraction is based mainly on forces from within a person's traits, the attraction is largely a projected ideal fantasy. This soon turns to disappointment.

Relational internalizations

Next is the influence of relational internalizations from infant attachment and later family dynamics. These are mainly the effects of the child's interaction with primary caregivers. An infant who started in life with an anxious, remote, or hostile mothering figure is likely to have love disturbances later in life. A secure attachment to a good enough mothering figure and family who gave the child love and a healthy sense of self and others are the interpersonal prerequisites to loving maturely.

Many people assume that it is the conscious memory that affects our behaviors. However, research has shown that the infants' implicit memory, which forms in the interactions with the mothering figure, remains unconscious and influential. This implicit memory affects individuals throughout their lifetime through their moods, capacity for closeness, and rewarding relationships (Fonagy, 2002; Walters, 2000).

The child's idealized image of the parenting figure(s) contributes to an idealization of the beloved. The person transfers the internalized, perceived image of the first love objects on to the new love object. It is hard to live up to a child's idealization of a parental figure who is godlike. The new love object will eventually become a disappointment if one is looking to replace an idealized parent. The new love object is often distorted based on the transferences from these relational internalizations. These transferences activate love, fear, and hate, all based on the quality of the original relationship with the parenting figures.

Beliefs

The next level is the beliefs from family, religion, cultural norms, and personal romantic experiences. These beliefs are often superstitious and irrational. We are good at rationalizing our irrational beliefs. The idealization of the beloved comes from sharing common ideals and the beloved fitting the family's or culture's notion of an ideal mate.

The relational internalizations of the parenting figures produce unconscious transferences to mates. These emotional transferences contribute to the formation of beliefs. It might take the form of, "Men are weak" (since my father was weak) or "Women are good mainly for sex" (since my mother was emotionally unreliable, I can only expect women to be sexually useful). These are neurotic remedies. They act to keep the person trapped in the self-defeating repetition of poor relationships.

For example, a neurotic remedy might be the belief that a controlling man is a strong man or that a sexually available woman will be empathically available. Both assumptions are wrong. A controlling man is, in fact, a weak man. A sexually available but unempathic woman is like the mother who is there only concretely in services, but not lovingly available.

In addition to the beliefs that come from transferences (the transference of feelings about parental figures on to current figures), there is also the cultural concept as to what is attractive in a mate.

Ayala Malach Pines (Pines, 1998, 2001; Pines & Zaidman, 2003) found that culture could modify evolutionary factors in what people find as attractive in a lover. In some cultures, a strong man means a physically strong man, while in other cultures, a strong man is defined by the abstract qualities of goodness and wisdom.

A person might have developed a belief about a potential mate based on his or her personal dating experiences. He might come to believe that women from certain religious backgrounds, ethnic groups, or even hair color will predict the success of the relationship. She might have come to believe, based on a past relationship, that men in certain professions are inherently unsuited. Most people, in fact, have ridiculous beliefs about others and relationships that they use to guide behavior (Harvey, 1989).

What does seem to matter is if couples share basic values and goals in life. In addition, the more individuals have beliefs and values that represent concern, integrity, fairness, and responsibility, the greater are the chances for a satisfying intimacy.

Current psychological context

The top level of the pyramid is the current psychological context. The overidealization of a lover at this level is caused by external conditions.

The time in a person's life or current stressful circumstances can produce conditions for an overidealization of another. People caught in disasters are vulnerable to fall in love. People who work together under stress, power differences, periods of neediness, and vulnerability can all help to create conditions of increased attraction. Dangerous and forbidden romances heighten passion. We all retain the thrill of wishing to do something naughty and rebellious. At the very least, the physiological state of arousal, be it erotic or fearful, can temporarily enhance infatuation (Stephan, 1971). People who met during a crisis, when they are vulnerable, or even on a roller coaster are more likely to become attracted to one another (Meston, 2003).

For example, the Stockholm Syndrome is a psychological reaction that leads to an attraction to a person holding one captive. The syndrome is named after a bank robbery in Stockholm in 1973. The bank robbers held bank employees hostage for about six days. This is also referred to as "capture-bonding," that is, the bond that can develop between captor and captive (Kuleshnyk, 1984).

A Swedish woman became so attracted to one of the bank robbers who held her hostage that she broke her engagement to her former lover and remained attached to her former captor while he served time in prison. This illustrates how a psychological context can create conditions for falling in love. The overidealization may be based on the current needs of the one and the power of the other to meet those needs. Our first loves—our parents—once had total control over us. This leaves us vulnerable to this type of transference. In addition, the woman might have had immature personality traits that allowed her to be vulnerable to capture-bonding.

As you move up the pyramid, you are moving from evolutionary history to current psychological context. Each level influences the others. For example, context eventually will affect natural selection and childhood relations, and cultural beliefs can modify instinctual species urges. All these levels in various combinations contribute to the irrationality of romantic love.

As people mature, the pyramid over time may begin to resemble a rectangle, with all the influences contributing more evenly. Instinctual urges diminish with age, traits may mature, childhood conflicts may become more metabolized with time, and life in the moment becomes more appreciated.

In any age, however, all these factors make up human motives:

$$\text{species traits} + \text{individual traits} + \\ \text{relational internalizations} + \text{beliefs} + \text{context.}$$

Table 1: How Each Level Contributes to Disturbed or Normal Love Relations.

The 5 Levels	Disturbed Love	Normal Love
Species Traits	Attraction is primarily based on primitive triggers	Attraction is not primarily based on primitive triggers
Individual Traits	Too much aggression, irrationality, egocentricity, unreliability, and defensiveness	A normal personality has the ability for sustained passion, concern, and commitment
Relational Internalizations	Attachment traumas, toxic internalizations of parenting figures cause fears, distortions, and provocations in intimacies	Secure attachment in infancy and a good enough childhood allows for a normal capacity for sustained love
Beliefs	Superstitious, irrational, unfair beliefs and concrete, selfish values	Strong sense of fairness and altruistic values
Current Context	Attraction is based on current fears or insecurities	Attraction is based on an appreciation of the good qualities of the other

What do you typically find attractive in a mate?

How much emphasis does attractiveness carry? Has it overridden important considerations?

Your personality traits came about by a combination of factors. You were born with a temperament based on biological inheritance. Then you were affected by the quality of attachment you had to your mothering figure. You unconsciously absorbed parts of your parents' personalities (both good and bad). How they treated you, the family dynamics, and societal experiences all helped to form your personality. These traits are unconscious most of the time.

Recognizing negative traits is difficult for anyone. You must have courage to do it. People who have self-acceptance feel comfortable with all sides of themselves. In order to grow and have good relations, you must see your faults without being defensive.

Look carefully over this list of traits. Honestly rate each of your traits with a 0 to 5 score.

None	Low		Medium		High
0	1	2	3	4	5

___ abandonment fears
___ addictions
___ aloofness
___ anger
___ anxiety
___ arrogance
___ being provocative
___ bitterness

__ control issues

__ cruel

__ defensiveness

__ demanding

__ depression

__ difficulty being understood by others

__ difficulty understanding others

__ being dramatic

__ easily bored

__ egocentricity

__ emptiness

__ entitlement feelings

__ fear of closeness

__ fear of commitment

__ fussiness

__ gloomy

__ guilt inducing

__ impatience

__ impulsivity

__ indecisiveness

__ inhibitions

__ insecurity

__ irresponsible

__ irritable

__ jealousy

__ laziness

__ moodiness

__ nagging

__ needing to be right

__ negativity

__ not fun

__ oppositional

__ overly dependent

__ overly sensitive

__ rigidity

__ seductiveness

__ seeing things in black and white

__ selfishness

__ stinginess

__ stubbornness

__ suspiciousness

__ too critical

__ unemotional

__ unfaithfulness

__ unreliability

__ untrustworthiness

__ other:_____

We all have faults. If you put "0" or "1" for most of the above, ask someone close to you if you are in denial or a candidate for sainthood. Go over your ratings with someone who will tell you the truth.

How do the above faults affect your relationships? Be honest. (Hint: Do not fool yourself. They have to affect your relationships!) If you are not sure, ask the same blunt person to tell you how they affect your relationships. A good friend will tell you when you are wrong and what your faults are because of concern for you. Your feelings might take a bruising, but you will get stronger. You can only grow with constructive feedback. The only standard is if the feedback is valid, fair, and constructive.

What faults can you improve on?

If appropriate, rate your partner, or if you are currently not in an intimate relationship, rate your last significant partner.

Look carefully over this list of traits. Honestly rate each trait with a 0 to 5 score.

None	Low		Medium		High
0	1	2	3	4	5

__abandonment fears
__addictions
__aloofness
__anger
__anxiety
__arrogance
__being provocative
__bitterness
__control issues
__cruel
__defensiveness
__demanding
__depressions
__difficulty being understood by others
__difficulty understanding others
__being dramatic
__easily bored
__egocentricity
__emptiness

__entitlement feelings
__fear of closeness
__fear of commitment
__fussiness
__gloomy
__guilt inducing
__impatience
__impulsivity
__indecisiveness
__inhibitions
__insecurity
__irresponsible
__irritable
__jealousy
__laziness
__moodiness
__nagging
__needing to be right
__negativity
__not fun
__oppositional
__overly dependent
__overly sensitive
__rigidity
__seductiveness
__seeing things in black and white
__selfishness
__stinginess
__stubbornness
__suspiciousness
__too critical
__unemotional

__unfaithfulness

__unreliability

__untrustworthiness

__other: _____

How much do your personality traits contribute to your relationship problems?

None	Low		Medium		High
0	1	2	3	4	5

How much do your partner's personality traits contribute to your relationship problems? Or if you are not currently in a relationship, how much did your former partner's personality traits contribute to your relationship problems?

None	Low		Medium		High
0	1	2	3	4	5

A person can unconsciously hurt others by:

1. Negative personality traits (such as hostility)
2. Defensiveness, such as denial or rationalizations (excuses)
3. Distortions, such as projections (falsely attributing to another your own problems) and negative transferences (transferring negative feelings about a parent on to your partner)

For a good relationship, it is important to know your faults, know when you are being defensive, and how your relationships with your parents in childhood influenced how you relate today.

How much did your relationships with your primary caregivers affect your intimacies?

None	Low		Medium		High
0	1	2	3	4	5

If you answered less than "medium," you may not understand that your relationship with your parents from infancy through childhood, for better or worse, had a major impact on your attractions and your capacity for intimacy. (The next chapter is devoted to the issue of parenting and later relations.)

You first loved as a child in a primitive, concrete manner based on your infantile needs.

Later you loved your parents less egocentrically, and finally, you love your parents as three-dimensional individuals with a healthy ambivalence. That is, you learn to love your parents as human beings with both faults and with good qualities.

You need to go through all the stages of love with your parents to love another wholly and maturely (psychoanalysts refer to this as resolving the Oedipal Complex). If your parents did not raise you through the normal developmental stages of learning to love and deal with anger and limits, you will later have a love disturbance. You might have the most passion for someone with a love disturbance.

How much of a healthy intimacy was modeled for you in childhood?

None	Low		Medium		High
0	1	2	3	4	5

How did your caregivers show emotions towards each other?

What kind of person did your family approve of when you were first dating?

How did these stereotypes contribute to what you found attractive during different stages of your life?

Considering your current psychological context, what needs, worries, opportunities, or limitations affect your attractions at this point in your life?

Please now take a second look at your responses. Look at yourself from the side—with more objectivity. How can your responses be deeper and more insightful? Could you be more honest, relevant, specific, and clear? Could you add anything more?

4

The Influence of Parenting on Later Love Relations

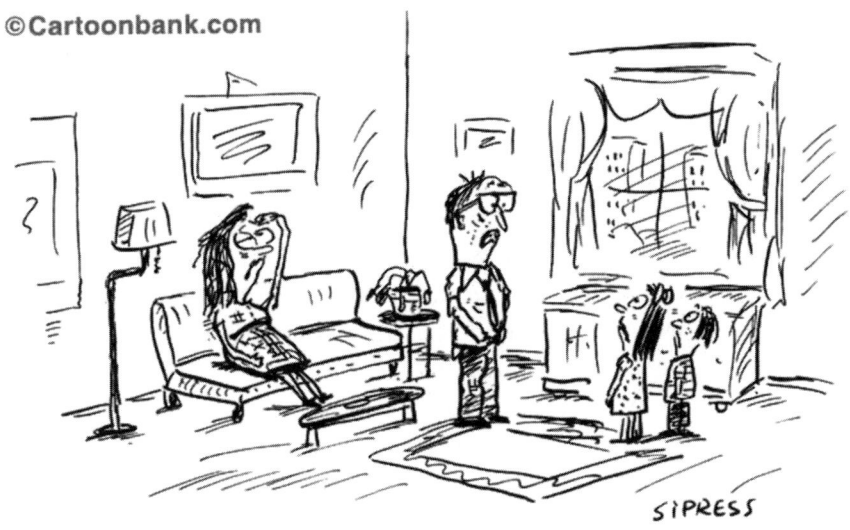

©Cartoonbank.com

SIPRESS

"Your mother and I are feeling overwhelmed, so you'll have to bring yourselves up."

Peter Fonagy (2002) studied the development of personality based on the mother's attachment style with her infant. Fonagy tested the attachment style of 96 women before they gave birth. He then tested the mothers' babies at 12 months of age. He found a 75% correspondence between the mothers' feelings about attachment and the children's personalities.

If the mother, before she gave birth, had Secure/Autonomous associations in her interview about attachment, then later the baby showed signs of a Secure attachment style of personality.

If the mother had Dismissing associations about attachment, then the baby showed signs of an Avoidant attachment (problems showing emotions).

If the mother had Preoccupied associations (easily emotionally upset) about attachment, then the baby showed signs of a Resistant or Ambivalent attachment (wary, distressed, angry, and passive).

If the mother had Unresolved/Disorganized associations (confusing and irrational) about attachment, then the baby showed signs of Disorganized/Disoriented attachment (disoriented, trancelike, and confused).

This and similar research illustrates how important interaction is from the very beginning of life in the shaping of personality and the capacity for later intimacy. The influence continues throughout childhood. The earlier the influences, the more powerful the effect is on personality. How do we know if the children's reactions to the parenting figure are lasting?

In a 20-year longitudinal study, researchers Walters, Merrick, Treboux, Crowell and Albersheim, (2000) looked at intimacy patterns in 50 young adults who were studied 20 years earlier as infants. Overall, 72% of the young adults received the same secure versus insecure attachment classification in their romantic relationships as they had in infancy.

That is, parents' attachment with their babies will affect their children's personalities and contribute to their children's love relations as adults. This effect is not based on conscious memory or thought; rather it is based on the mothering figure affecting the development of the child's right brain's emotional and relational ability to regulate affects[1], self-sooth, form concepts of the self and others, and capacity to love (Schore, 1994).

In addition to attachment in infancy, Walters et al. also found that other negative life experiences also affected the type of adult love relations, such as: loss of a parent, parental divorce, life-threatening illness of a parent or the child, parental psychiatric disorder, and physical or sexual abuse by a family member.

---

[1]Psychologists commonly use the word "affects" for feelings, emotions and moods.

While the infant research used mothers, gender is not the issue (which is why we use terms like, "mothering figure," "parenting figure," or "primary caregiver"). Children benefit from having parents in the roles of "mothering" and "fathering." The mothering role is one of nurturance and protection. The fathering role has powerful implications to the development of personality in the child. The father figure pulls the child out of the dependent attachment to the mother and toughens the child for the outside world. The father affects self-esteem, confidence, achievement, motivation, and the ability to live within limits with discipline (Cath, 1982).

As we move from the pre-Oedipal period (the dyad of the infant and mothering figure), we move to the Oedipal family triad. The resolution of the Oedipal triad is necessary for learning to love outside a closed dyad. That is, the mother and father figures, as a team, help the child learn to share love. In adult life, the couple must learn to negotiate with the demands of others (children, parents, friends, and the world of work). This will be difficult if, as children, they did not have to share their love for a parent with another.

Children need to learn to negotiate needs and not feel entitled to having needs met. Children need to share their love objects, develop a sense of "good enough," and have appreciation. Children also need to learn to express their basic instincts (sexuality and aggression) in a constructive manner. If the basic Oedipal issues of managing sexuality, aggression, limits, and sharing are not resolved, there will be love disturbances.

The relationships with parents are crucial in personality development and ability to relate to others. Bradley (1974) studied 205 families who were seeking services for psychological problems for their children. They found a significant relationship between the personalities of both the mother and the father as measured by the MMPI (an objective test of psychopathology). Each of the parent's scores in psychopathology related to disturbances in their children.

We recreate our childhood attachments, traumas, and conflicts in our intimate relationships. Our childhood perceptions of our parents, as idealized gods or as tormenting demons, became internal gyroscopes orienting us to lovers who evoke similar emotions in us. If we imprinted on a tormenting parent, then a tormenting lover will be exciting and a kind lover will seem boring. We can repeat our childhood relationships by unconsciously picking a lover who evokes similar emotions from childhood, or we can provoke or distort our lover in order to repeat an intimacy pattern. (I will discuss this important unconscious enactment later on.)

Our original family intimacies became our "normal." Sometimes we are just confused as to how to even recognize or react to emotional problems in a lover if dysfunctional relationships have been so much of our childhood experiences. The love drama is repeated over and over and sometimes the roles are interchangeable. If our lover is not the tormentor, then we become the tormentor. (Of course, this is unconscious and rationalized.) Nevertheless, the love drama is the same, moving towards the same outcome. If our primary caregivers were negligent or traumatizing, you can predict that the outcomes of our later passions will tend to produce the same emotions we had in childhood.

Some people with traumatic childhoods do not seem to act out their dramas; rather they internalize it. They are more likely to suffer anxiety and depression since their internal relational world is filled with anger, fear, and hurt.

If we had good enough parents and have a secure identity, then romantic love usually evolves into lasting love. Many people are not so lucky. Many of us need to work hard to love wisely. The only way we know to alter a love disturbance is through emotional insight in the context of a healthy intimacy (example: insight psychotherapy).

Our core personality is formed by our attachments in early childhood while the (right) brain is still forming. This core continues to form throughout our childhood. We unconsciously try to repeat the patterns of attachments in our current love relations. If there are childhood traumas with loss, aggression, neglect, impingement, or exploitation, this attachment drama becomes part of the self. This drama repeats itself in future attachments to achieve the same emotional result as in childhood. If there was conflict with a parent, so then there will be conflict with our current love. When we enter into intimacy, we regress and repeat our unconscious emotional past without realizing it.

Every person in the family system exerts an influence on each other's behaviors. Our roles in our family helped to keep the family emotionally operating. We might have been in the role of a rescuer, scapegoat, or messiah, depending on the needs of the family system. These roles also become part of our unconscious drama that we enact in our intimacies (Gordon, 1982). If there was conflict in the family system, then the conflict will become part of the child's personality system.

Each child's temperament interacts with the family system. Some children are naturally resilient, and they are less affected by traumas. The original family system—that is, our parents' personalities, their relationship, how they treated us, and our temperament— all come together in forming the implicit (unconscious) personality (Gordon, 2005).

Our unconscious does not perceive any new love as new, but rather in terms of our first loves as children. We can repeat the past by:

1. Picking someone with similar qualities of a parent (example: you have the most passion for a lover who is as critical as your parent is);
2. Unconsciously provoking the partner into acting like the parent figure (example: you provoke your lover's criticism by acting as a child);
3. Distorting the perception of the partner to seem like the parent (example: you misperceive your partner as being unfairly critical).

We do any or all of these—picking, provoking, and distorting— in order to repeat unconsciously the imprinting and traumas (Gordon, 1998). In love, we have the urge to return to our unresolved issues.

Must we be slaves to these patterns? No. Insight can disrupt self-defeating patterns. I hope this workbook will provide you with some insights to help you disrupt self-defeating patterns.

We can make a distinction when we are upset between how much of our feelings are coming from our own issues and how much are attributable to the other person. If we reflect on these insights rather than act out, our intimacies might not become the toxic waste dump for our unresolved conflicts. Defensive people try not to think about the past or their patterns, but unconsciously act out their problems in their relationships.

People often take out on their partner the unresolved anger and fears they had for a parent. With this imagined revenging, they never detoxify the past, but only reinforce it. They do not learn and grow to love maturely.

Insight into these unconscious, self-defeating patterns is not sufficient to detoxify them. It is only a start. However, insight can do damage control. It can help you understand the causes of the interpersonal problems and have remorse without defensiveness. It might even help to prevent the actual expression of provocative behavior. You might be better able to understand your partner and know how to react without making things worse.

Now let us now get specific. Write as honestly as you can. Go deeper than you might in causal thought or conversation. Consider your relationship with a parent during your childhood and not later on. If there was no relationship with a parent, state how that might have affected you. By "mother," I mean "primary mothering figure." By "father," I mean "primary fathering figure."

Feel free to answer any way that helps you understand how you were raised. Perhaps, a stepparent had influence on you during your critical period of personality development (from birth to about ten years old). Use all the parental figures that had influence on you.

It will not be easy to answer some of these questions. The earliest experiences of childhood will not be in conscious memory. They are stored in an implicit memory. In later childhood, the retrievable memories may be repressed or distorted. The only way to have an educated guess about your relevant childhood history is:

1. By logical inference; for example, if your mother had always been warm, empathic, and easygoing, she was probably like that in your early childhood. Similarly, if your father has always been egocentric and uninvolved, he was likely that

way in your childhood. In addition, parents might have had children when they were young and immature. Later they often mature; however, most deep-seated personality traits do not change.

2. By reliable reports from others; for example, a patient in psychotherapy reports that a few months before he was born, his sister died. His mother was in a major depression during his infancy. Another patient was in an orphanage for the first 18 months of her life. Neither is able to remember these circumstances. Both had little emotional contact in their first months of life. Both have serious problems with intimacy based on these infantile traumas. These histories, though not remembered, have been validated by others.

3. Before language, the child's experiences are stored in the physiology of the body and in the emotions. We express those experiences in our diseases and in our intimacies. Language acquisition in childhood helps with the recall of some memories. However, the child's subjectivity, fantasies, and temperament all contribute to the misperception of events. We can recall both our emotional history and actual history. However, our defense mechanisms help to regulate anxiety. If the memories could threaten our self-esteem or produce too much anxiety, then the memories could become repressed and distorted. Nevertheless, we all retain some ability to remember the past.

Now try your best. Be honest, clear, to the point, and complete. If you are not sure about your past, ask someone who will tell you.

Which of your parents was more empathic, affectionate, involved, and understanding in your childhood?

___ Mother   ___ Father   ___ Neither   ___ Both equally

Other:

When you were a child, how happy were your parents with one another?

Not	Low		Medium		Very Happy
0	1	2	3	4	5

How much conflict was in their relationship?

None	Low		Medium		High
0	1	2	3	4	5

Did your parents ever separate during your childhood?

___ Yes   ___ No

If you answered "Yes," then what age were you? (If they separated more than once, put your ages when it occurred.)

Did your parents ever divorce?

___ Yes   ___ No

If you answered "Yes," then what age were you?

What was the nature of your parent's relationship(s) that you observed as a child?

Overall, how much trauma, losses, abuse, or neglect did you have in your childhood?

None	Low		Medium		High
0	1	2	3	4	5

What were they? What hurts and disappointments have affected you?

What are the current triggers that you react to because of your past?

How much affection did your mother show you?

None	Low		Medium		High
0	1	2	3	4	5

How did she show it?

How does this affect your current intimacies?

How much affection did your father show you?

None	Low		Medium		High
0	1	2	3	4	5

How did he show it?

How does this affect your current intimacies?

How well did your mother understand your innermost feelings?

None	Low		Medium		High
0	1	2	3	4	5

How does this affect your current intimacies?

How well did your father understand your innermost feelings?

None	Low		Medium		High
0	1	2	3	4	5

How does this affect your current intimacies?

How much anger did your mother have?

None	Low		Medium		High
0	1	2	3	4	5

How did it come out?

How does this affect your current intimacies?

How much anger did your father have?

None	Low		Medium		High
0	1	2	3	4	5

How did it come out?

How does this affect your current intimacies?

How well did each of your parents deal with the issue of sexuality?

Mother:

Badly	Low		Medium		Very Well
0	1	2	3	4	5

Father:

Badly	Low		Medium		Very Well
0	1	2	3	4	5

How does this affect your current intimacies?

How well did each of your parents deal with boundaries and privacy?

Mother:

Badly	Low		Medium		Very Well
0	1	2	3	4	5

Father:

Badly	Low		Medium		Very Well
0	1	2	3	4	5

How does this affect your current intimacies?

How much were you included in your mother's life?

None	Low		Medium		High
0	1	2	3	4	5

How does this affect your current intimacies?

How much were you included in your father's life?

None	Low		Medium		High
0	1	2	3	4	5

How does this affect your current intimacies?

How well did your parents teach you values and ethics?

None	Low		Medium		High
0	1	2	3	4	5

How fair were your parents with you?

Not	Low		Medium		High
0	1	2	3	4	5

How does this affect your current intimacies?

How comfortable did you feel with your mother?

None	Low		Medium		High
0	1	2	3	4	5

How does this affect your current intimacies?

How comfortable did you feel with your father?

None	Low		Medium		High
0	1	2	3	4	5

How does this affect your current intimacies?

Now look at the self-esteem of your parents. By self-esteem, I do not mean narcissism. I mean a comfortable self-acceptance.

What was the self-esteem of your mother?

None	Low		Medium		High
0	1	2	3	4	5

How did her self-esteem affect you?

What was the self-esteem of your father?

None	Low		Medium		High
0	1	2	3	4	5

How did his self-esteem affect you?

How would you rate your self-esteem?

None	Low		Medium		High
0	1	2	3	4	5

How would you rate the self-esteem of your partner? (Or if not in a current relationship, your last partner.)

None	Low		Medium		High
0	1	2	3	4	5

How defensive was your mother during your childhood?

None	Low		Medium		High
0	1	2	3	4	5

How defensive was your father during your childhood?

None   Low   Medium   High
0   1   2   3   4   5

How did their degree of defensiveness affect you? How does this affect your current intimacies?

How defensive is your partner (or if not in a current relationship, your last partner)?

None   Low   Medium   High
0   1   2   3   4   5

How well did your mother support and encourage your independence?

None   Low   Medium   High
0   1   2   3   4   5

How well did your father support and encourage your independence?

None	Low		Medium		High
0	1	2	3	4	5

How does this affect your current intimacies?

How did either of your parents encourage your success?

Remember rating your faults and those of a significant other? Now rate each of your parents. You may redefine "Mother" and "Father" if you grew up in a nontraditional home.

Look carefully over this list of traits. Rate each trait with a 0 to 5 score for both your mother (M) and your father (F).

None	Low		Medium		High
0	1	2	3	4	5

M   **F**

____   ____ abandonment fears
____   ____ addictions
____   ____ aloofness
____   ____ anger
____   ____ anxiety
____   ____ arrogance
____   ____ being provocative
____   ____ bitterness
____   ____ control issues
____   ____ cruel
____   ____ defensiveness
____   ____ demanding
____   ____ depressions
____   ____ difficulty being understood by others
____   ____ difficulty understanding others
____   ____ being dramatic
____   ____ easily bored
____   ____ egocentricity
____   ____ emptiness
____   ____ entitlement feelings
____   ____ fear of closeness
____   ____ fear of commitment

____   ____ fussiness

____   ____ gloomy

____   ____ guilt inducing

____   ____ impatience

____   ____ impulsivity

____   ____ indecisiveness

____   ____ inhibitions

____   ____ insecurity

____   ____ irresponsible

____   ____ irritable

____   ____ jealousy

____   ____ laziness

____   ____ moodiness

____   ____ nagging

____   ____ needing to be right

____   ____ negativity

____   ____ not fun

____   ____ oppositional

____   ____ overly dependent

____   ____ overly sensitive

____   ____ rigidity

____   ____ seductiveness

____   ____ seeing things in black and white

____   ____ selfishness

____   ____ stinginess

____   ____ stubbornness

____   ____ suspiciousness

____   ____ too critical

____   ____ unemotional

____   ____ unfaithfulness

____   ____ unreliability

____   ____ untrustworthiness

____   ____ other:_____

To what extent were you ever encouraged to side with a parent?

None	Low		Medium		High
0	1	2	3	4	5

Why?

To what extent were you ever encouraged to reject a parent?

Never	Low		Medium		High
0	1	2	3	4	5

What is the longest time you did not speak to a parent because of a conflict? Put the amount of time (days, weeks, months, years).

_____

(Example: 5 days or 5 years; make sure to put in numbers)

Have you ever stopped a relationship with a parent?

___ Yes   ___ No

Why?

Have you ever stopped a relationship with a parent after your parents divorced?

___ Yes   ___ No   ___ NA (Not Applicable)

Why?

How does this affect your current intimacies?

Were you too close to a parent?

___ Yes   ___ No

If yes, which one?

How does this affect your current intimacies?

What was your role within your family of origin (examples: rescuer, scapegoat, strong one, weak one, crazy one, invisible, golden child, etc.)?

How does that role continue to express itself in your current relationship(s)?

How did other members of your family affect you and your current intimacies?

Who was the most positive role model of your childhood and why?

Our relational internalizations of our primary caregivers are stored in our unconscious and have a powerful affect on our love relations. Children require a loving, safe, and supportive relationship with parents to develop normally. If a child experiences being used in the middle of parent's conflicts or is turned against a parent, this will affect the development of love relations. Here is an except from the my book, *An Expert Look at Love, Intimacy and Personal Growth* (Gordon, 2006d).

> I have found that those people who have been alienated against a parent in childhood will have love disturbances. If they are to have a chance at healthy relationships, they will need to work through their love dramas in the therapeutic-committed intimacy with the therapist.
> Many nonanalytically trained individuals, not working with unconscious distortions, take at face value the patient's complaints and memories, and thereby reinforce the alienation and the love disturbances. Working with only the conscious is too superficial to get to the damage from early pathological attachment. Patients have a hard time putting into language all that they felt and parents implied or acted out. A disturbed parent uses language to rationalize and to distort reality. Interpretations can make sense out of confused emotions. The therapy also needs to be a holding environment with a good container. The therapeutic relationship must be long and intense to achieve the necessary personal growth . . .

Your temperament and your childhood relationships with parents are perhaps the most powerful determinates of the success of your relationships. You had no control over these things. However, be optimistic. The more you have insight about these parts of you, the more you can be in control and not let things get out of hand.

Even if you are not in insight psychotherapy, you can begin to use insight from what you are learning here. That is the point of this workbook. I want to help you understand and control any problems that inevitably pop out in intimacy. Think about the traits in your parents that you hate to admit that comes out in your relationships. Be aware of them. Contain them. Do reality testing. Self-sooth. Use insight. Be constructive. I will discuss these steps later on. Now let us try to better understand this thing called "Romantic Love."

5

What Is Romantic Love?

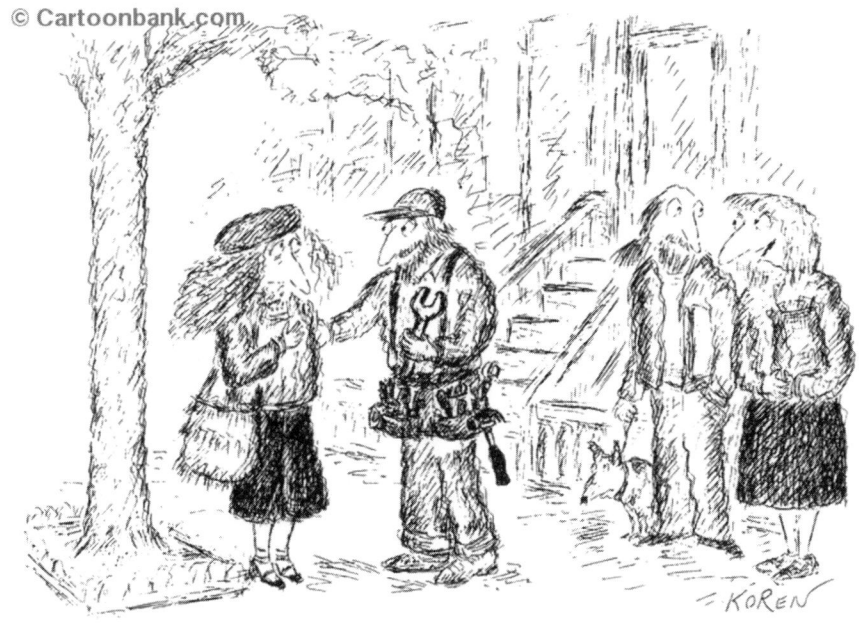

"They're a perfect match—she's high-maintenance, and he can fix anything."

Romantic love is a temporary delusional state of overidealization for another. It is nature's way to trick us into a reproductive mood for the survival of the species. Instinctively, infatuation only lasts from about two minutes to two years, long enough for the likelihood of offspring. Of course, this temporary idealizing delusion can lead to a great deal of personal embarrassment and loss of significant resources in a divorce.

Sometimes romantic love can last for years, or even a lifetime. This can happen when there is a lack of significant time together. These conditions can keep the idealized fantasy of the beloved protected from the practical demands of reality and the wearing down from negative personality traits.

Romantic love can also last when couples know how to be intimate and remain caring. They do not feel entitled to everlasting love. They work at it and succeed.

Let us first explore what romantic love is.

Romantic love is the combination of passion and intimacy. Passion is the fuel of romantic love. Passion by its nature is obsessive and addictive. There are several reasons for this. When you feel "chemistry" for someone, actual changes in your brain chemistry occur. You have increased levels of dopamine and norepinephrine and decreased levels of serotonin in your brain (Fisher 2000). This is related to states of euphoria and obsessionalism. This biological state of love addiction may be a product of natural selection in that it increases the likelihood of reproduction.

Added to this biochemical idealization is the psychological idealization of the lover. The lover can be a projection of one's ideal self or the transference from the idealized parental image. Everyone has an unconscious ideal self left over from childhood. In narcissistic personalities, the ideal self is grandiose and becomes the core of personality. However, even in those with low self-esteem, there is an ideal self. They feel that they can never live up to their ideal self and they therefore feel inferior.

Love based on grandiose projections tends to be more disturbed than those loves based on transference. Projections are primitive distortions of reality. Projections are a confusion of where the self-boundary ends and the other boundary begins. Transferences are also distortions of another, but with some sense of boundary and reality.

With infatuation, an overidealization is projected or transferred onto a potential mate. This primitive idealization is unconsciously placed onto the beloved, whether the love is earned or not. One is never addicted to a real person. One is only addicted to the object of the idealization.

There is always some idealization in love. In normal love, the idealization has more basis in the real qualities of the beloved than in subjective, erotic fantasy or one's personal needs. The more a person is looking to someone else to fill the empty spaces of one's self, the more that person will become dependent on an idealized love. A person with a weak sense of self looks for love to provide contentment. The lover is expected to provide the person with happiness and unconditional love. This is a child's notion of love.

Passion can stay alive in a healthy intimacy as long as there is just the right amount of aggression. Too much aggression kills love. Too little aggression kills passion. Sublimating passion (expressing passion in a creative, nonharmful manner) in humor, teasing, and erotic playfulness helps it stay alive.

Typically, how long does romantic love last for you? Why?

6

What Are the Stages of Romantic Love?

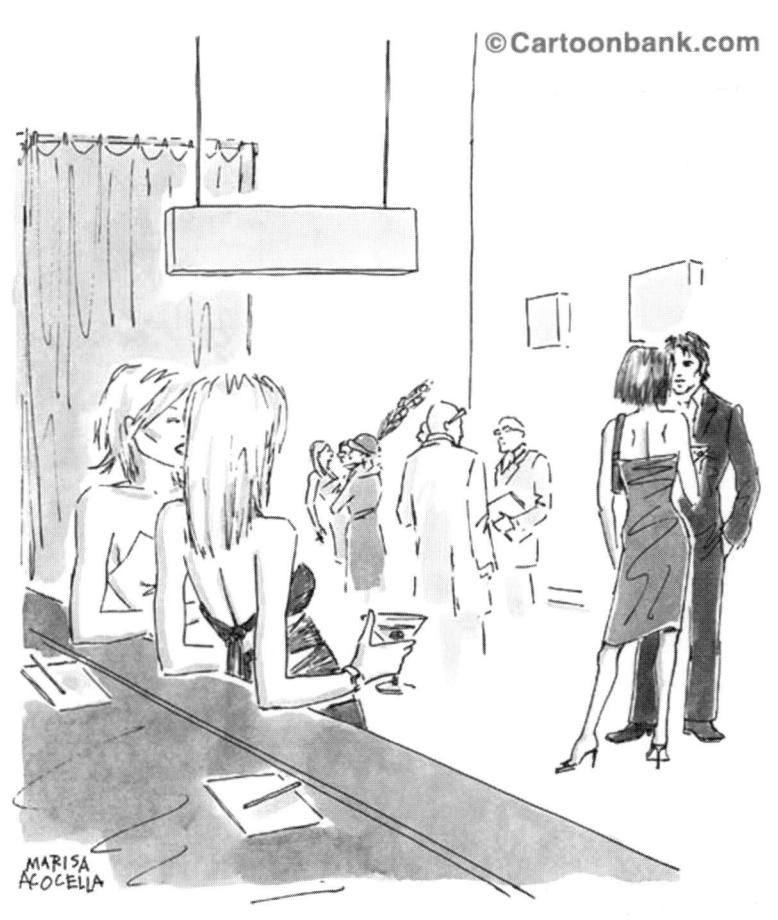

©Cartoonbank.com

MARISA
ACOCELLA

"He's your type—gorgeous, successful, and totally unavailable."

Avner Ziv's (1993) research based on his interviews with single and married men and women suggests four stages of romantic love:

1. The Attraction stage of romantic love is a reaction to concrete triggers, mainly physical attraction.

2. In the Examination stage of romantic love, people take a closer look at the surface facts. They see how well they match in such areas as intelligence, interests, values and emotional compatibility and comfort. However, both individuals are in the stage of still "selling" themselves. They are likely to exaggerate their positive features and how much they have in common.

3. The Self-Revealing stage is a deeper look at personality including the negative features. It is at this stage intimacy is created.

4. The Mutual Expectation stage is how well the relationship works in dealing with the practical tasks of life. This includes meeting expectations and satisfying needs in the economic, emotional, social and sexual areas.

What stages did you go through? What were they like? What usually happens in each stage? Why?

The Attraction stage

The Examination stage

The Self-Revealing stage

The Mutual Expectation stage

7

What Are Disturbed Love Relations?

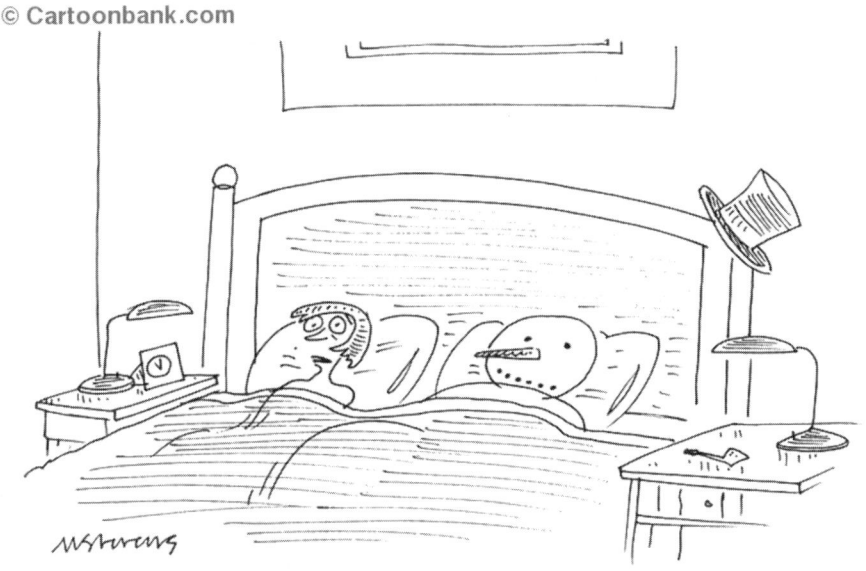

"You'll be gone in the morning, just like all the others."

Otto Kernberg (1974) wrote of two basic love disturbances found in the most psychologically primitive of individuals:

1. The inability to fall in love
2. The inability to remain in love

Salman Akhtar (1999) added three more love disturbances:

3. The tendency to fall in love with the "wrong" kinds of people
4. The inability to fall out of love
5. The inability to feel loved

The most severe form of love disturbance is the inability to fall in love. In order to fall in love, some degree of idealization or over-valuing is necessary. In normal love, the idealization is primarily based on an appreciation of the real qualities of the beloved. In pathological cases, the idealization is mainly delusional with an equal but opposite devaluation lurking beneath. However, people who cannot fall in love at all either cannot feel an idealization of another or the idealization is a fickle and fleeting fantasy.

Individuals may have problems falling in love because:

1. They are too egocentric. They lack the capacity to love another.
2. They dread closeness since closeness is associated with the destruction of their fragile psychological world.

The next level of disturbance is when a person can fall in love but cannot remain in love. Personalities that fall into this category have the capacity for idealization and erotic desire. They unconsciously seek a magical love that is worthy of their grandiose self and also a rescuer that is transformational. However, they experience a great deal of hostility when the idealized love object does not live up to the hoped for magical transformation. They may become obsessed with deficiencies in the love object. They often unconsciously fear that intimacy will reveal that they are a fraud and may project this onto the love object and come to see the formally idealized lover as a fraud. A cycle of idealization and devaluation of the other moves the person in and out of closeness. There is no true intimacy with a real person. Their love is like a child's fantasy. They fall in love with a fantasy and then punish the real person for not obeying the fantasy.

Individuals may evolve from not being able to fall in love, to being able to fall in love but not remain in love. They might fall in love with the "wrong people" in service to their unconscious need to not remain in love.

About a hundred years ago, Freud wrote a paper, "A Special Type of Object Made by Men" (1910a). Freud wrote of the "rescue complex" and the "whore/Madonna split." Freud wrote " . . . the desire they express to 'rescue' the beloved . . . the libido has dwelt so long in its attachment to the mother . . . that the maternal characteristics remain stamped on the love-objects chosen later . . . the idea of 'rescue' actually has a significance and history of its own and is an independent derivative of the mother-complex, or more correctly, of the parental complex . . ."

Freud was describing the sexual excitement of falling in love with the wrong sort of person, since that love object represented a rebellion against the family. The unconscious love drama also represents a rescuing of a parental figure from the other parent. There is often a split between sexuality and being a "good" person. This might be the result of the parent-child relationship not dealing with sexuality in a healthy manner. The child might have not been able to see the parent as both sexual and good. When this happens, the erotic desire becomes greater toward a "wrong" kind of person.

The next love disturbance is the inability to fall out of love. Most people would fall out of love when it is necessary to do so. Salman Akhtar felt that normally if love is unrequited or toxic, the love diminishes and there is a normal grieving process. However, individuals with an immature personality structure and obsessional features do the opposite and intensify their attachment when love is not reciprocated. They are highly invested in their sadomasochistic needs. They refuse to accept limits that should have been resolved with the Oedipal situation. In other words, children need to learn that they cannot possess and control the love object to feel secure and have a sense of worth. They cannot own the parent. They must deal with limits and loss and learn from it.

Finally, there are people who can give love, but feel uncomfortable receiving love. Such people may have been too hurt and feel safer as the giver than as the receiver. According to Akhtar, people who have problems with being loved have difficulty with renouncing masochism, dealing with "good enough," loss, and their own unconscious aggression.

Which love disturbances are problems for you?

The inability to fall in love

None	Low		Medium		High
0	1	2	3	4	5

The inability to remain in love

None	Low		Medium		High
0	1	2	3	4	5

The tendency to fall in love with the "wrong" kinds of people

None	Low		Medium		High
0	1	2	3	4	5

The inability to fall out of love

None	Low		Medium		High
0	1	2	3	4	5

The inability to feel loved

None	Low		Medium		High
0	1	2	3	4	5

If applicable, which love disturbances are problems for your partner? (Or if not in a current relationship, your last partner.)

The inability to fall in love

None	Low		Medium		High
0	1	2	3	4	5

The inability to remain in love

None	Low		Medium		High
0	1	2	3	4	5

The tendency to fall in love with the "wrong" kinds of people

None	Low		Medium		High
0	1	2	3	4	5

The inability to fall out of love

None	Low		Medium		High
0	1	2	3	4	5

The inability to feel loved

None	Low		Medium		High
0	1	2	3	4	5

What you can do

You can manage love disturbances with containment, reality testing, insight, self-soothing, and constructive action.

Containment requires not acting out tensions, not denying or projecting tensions, but tolerating them until they are constructively resolved. A child needs a mothering figure to contain the child's emotions. Children who had mothers who were good emotion containers can later tolerate stress well. A patient often needs a psychotherapist to be a good container of the patient's emotions. Eventually, the patient learns to contain and tolerate his or her own emotions without dumping them into someone else. For example, "I know that I am in a bad mood. I can contain it until I can sooth myself and get some insight." Or, "I know she is in a bad mood and needs me to listen. She needs me to be a good container of her emotions right now."

Reality testing is the weighting of evidence in objective reality, as opposed to making assumptions based on feelings, guesses, and projections. For example, "I'm glad I did some reality testing. I thought about my history with him, I talked with people who know him well, and his responses were consistent and plausible. There is no objective evidence for my suspicions. I must have been wrong, because I was so afraid." (This example is for teaching purposes. In reality, the process is more casual.)

Insight means seeing the underlying or unconscious reasons for doing something irrational. Instead of rationalizing (making rational sounding excuses), insight helps you to see how and why you are setting yourself up. You can use insight into your issues or your partner's issues to help you problem solve conflicts. Insight can help you see the problems more deeply and resolve them more constructively. You can grow by learning from your mistakes when you use insight versus being defensive.

Self-soothing can be at a superficial level and it can be at a deep level. Superficial self-soothing can be using distractions (time-out), calming techniques (counting to ten, listening to music, slow, mindful breathing), or cognitive affirmations ("so what?", "no one is perfect"). For example, after a fight, superficial self-soothing could be, "So what if he doesn't like my cooking? No one is perfect. I'll calm down and listen to some music for a while."

Ideally, self-soothing is combined with insight so that it is deeper, more effective, and can lead to personal growth. With insight, you can self-sooth by pin-pointing the specific ways that you upset yourself or make things worse. For example, insightful self-soothing could be, "I know I overreacted to this trigger because it is an issue for me. It is not as bad as I made it out to be."

Constructive action can follow from reality testing and insightful self-soothing. For example, "Before I act out anymore (containment), I wonder why I am so sensitive about his not liking my cooking. He was not mean about it. He was just honest (reality testing). I am overreacting because I could never please my father. It reminded me of how I used to feel in my childhood (insight). Besides, I know he hates liver (reality testing). Why did I make it for him? I think I might have provoked him so I could feel as I did with my father (insight). It helps to understand what happened. I feel better figuring this out (self-soothing). I will go over to him and share with him why I provoked him and apologize for starting a fight about this (corrective action)."

Think of a conflict you had with your partner (or with someone in the past) and to what degree you used containment, reality testing, insight, self-soothing, and constructive action. Write how you might have used containment, reality testing, insight, self-soothing, and constructive action better.

Containment

Reality Testing

Insight

Self-Soothing

Constructive Action

8

How Temperaments
Affect Love Relations

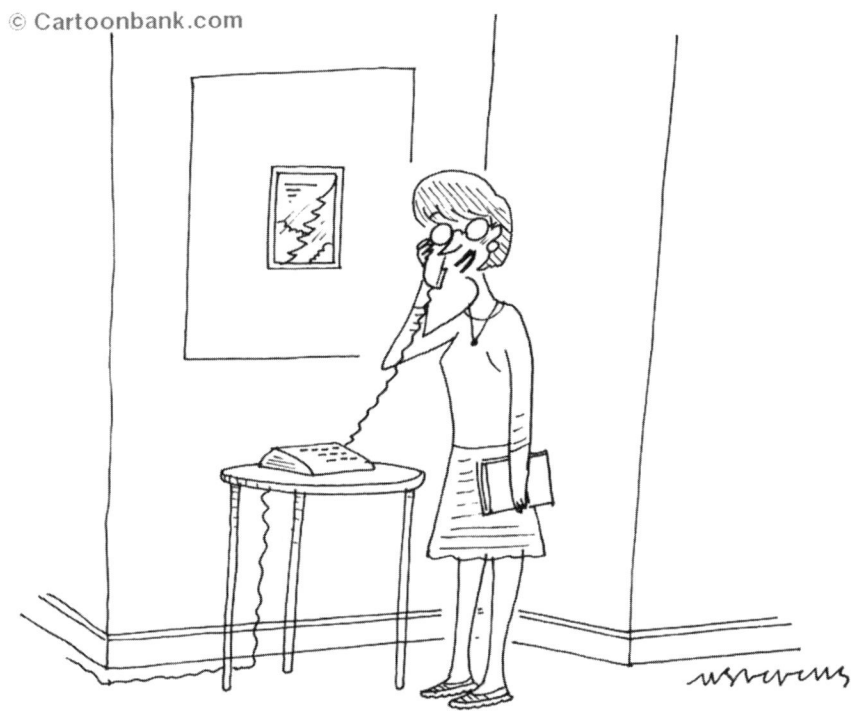

"I'd <u>love</u> to, but that's my Women's Rage Workshop night."

Healthy ambivalence and a whole person perception

How we see each other is based on the reality of the person and on our own projections and transferences. The more disturbed the person, the more others become objects of a person's subjective distortions. The love and hate may become a subjective acting out of an unconscious drama. The erotic stimulation may not be for a whole person, but a body surface or part or article of clothing as with perversions, or to a substance or drugs as in an addictive disorder.

If the idealization of a beloved is based mainly in immature projections and transferences, the idealization can quickly switch to devaluation and persecutory hate. An immature personality views an object of dependency based on needs and moods and not on the enduring qualities of the person.

A mature person can love with a healthy ambivalence. A person with a healthy ambivalence tolerates the normal fluctuations of mood within the total enduring bond of the relationship. The love and hate are not split into opposing emotions that redefine the significant other. The beloved does not become a devil or angel according to one's moods.

A person with a healthy ambivalent love can appreciate the actual qualities and complex nature of the other person, regardless of needs and emotions. A person with an immature personality swings between feeling grandiosity and deflation of the self, and idealization and devaluation of the other.

A mature person has both self-love and other-love, based on an awareness of both assets and liabilities that are blended together into a cohesive self-concept and concept of the other.

Immature people cannot tolerate the ambiguity of emotional grays, but go to black or white perceptions and evaluations. This leads to idealizations and devaluations that swing the intimacy beyond the tolerance of their centrifugal force.

The intensity of an immature person's idealized love can look like the stuff of a great and lasting love. It is not. The intensity of love is not a measure of its maturity. However, initially such intensity can be very appealing.

Most people avoid insight and seek an ideal love with a magical hero or heroine (Bergmann, 1982; Freud, 1914/1957). Falling in love is a return to the emotions of infancy when we felt a magical symbiosis with an idealized caregiver. In childhood, our love matures with the interaction of healthy parents. With the continuing lessons of love that we can learn in a healthy family, we later can fall in love with a realistic appreciation of the beloved. With too much emotional trauma, an infantile notion of a magical love becomes fixated and is repeated in adult love relations. Mature love requires the idealization of truth; immature love requires the idealization of love itself.

The three levels of personality organization

Now let us look at what constitutes a mature versus immature personality. There are seven standards recommended by the Psychodynamic Diagnostic Manual (PDM, 2006) to measure an individual's level of maturity.

1. A stable identity—a realistic and integrated sense of self
2. The capacity for stable, satisfying intimacy
3. Affect tolerance—ability to experience and tolerate age appropriate emotions
4. Affect regulation—ability to experience and express emotions appropriately
5. A mature ethical and value system
6. Good reality testing
7. Good ability to handle stress and to be resilient

The PDM classifies three main levels of personality structure or organization. The healthy level (absence of a personality disorder) is characterized by the person's overall ability to handle the stress and challenges of life. The healthy person is mainly healthy. However, they could develop some symptoms under stress. They have a stable identity and a good capacity for affect regulation and tolerance, objectivity, remorse, and intimacy.

People at the neurotic level of personality organization use the higher-level defenses such as repression (more on defensive style in the next chapter). The people at the neurotic level have problems in only certain areas of their lives. They usually have good relationships and intimacies. However, they can become overwhelmed by anxiety, depression, phobias, somatizations (psychologically involved physical problems), guilt, and inhibitions. They tend to have good contact with reality.

People at the borderline level of personality organization favor the primitive defenses such as denial, splitting, and projective identification. These defenses distort and deny reality and cause a great deal of interpersonal problems. Individuals at the borderline level of personality organization have recurrent interpersonal problems. They have problems with stable emotions and intimacies. They can be moody, vulnerable, dependent, impulsive, addiction prone, self-harming, and hostile. They have problems with identity and boundaries. They often externalize blame and do not see how they contribute to their problems.

Someone with a borderline personality organization can have several types of personality disorders, i.e. Schizoid, Paranoid, Psychopathic, Narcissistic, Sadistic, Masochistic Depressive, Somatizing, Dependent, Phobic, Anxious, Obsessive-Compulsive, Hysterical, Dissociative, or Mixed Personality Disorder. The more borderline traits a person has, the more these personality disorders are a problem in relationships.

For example, egocentricity characterizes the Narcissistic Personality Disorder. The person may have grandiosity and act haughty and arrogant. They often have feelings of being special, only understandable to special, privileged people. They often have a need for excessive admiration and have a sense of entitlement, in that they expect special treatment from others. However, they often feel infringed upon when similar demands are placed on them. They are often exploitive, have problems with empathy, and are unable or unwilling to recognize the feelings and needs of others. They often feel envy and accuse others of envying them. People with a Narcissistic Personality Disorder are often overly concerned with power, success, beauty, or ideal love.

If the Narcissistic disorder is within a borderline personality organization, then there are more intense emotions and tumultuous intimacy. There is usually a history of unstable interpersonal relationships. Their intimacies constantly alternate between idealization and devaluation. One moment they cannot live without their love object, and the next moment, the love object is seen as persecutory and is demonized and devalued. They suffer from an unstable self-image. They often do not really feel that they have a distinct identity, and they suffer from low self-esteem. They are often impulsive, use bad judgment, and are frequently in a state of confusion. Depression is a problem and may include suicidal thoughts and/or behaviors. There is emotional instability and moodiness, with periods of intense anxiety, agitation, and irritability. They frequently have feelings of inner emptiness with inappropriate, intense anger and can have paranoid thoughts.

If the borderline personality organization is mixed with a Masochistic Personality Disorder, the person is a perpetual victim. They constantly put themselves in situations where they are injured in one fashion or another. They get others to hurt them. They have frequent accidents. They provoke and engage in situations where they can end up hurt, both emotionally and physically.

If a person's identity is unstable, then that person's perceptions of others will be unstable. The person will love only parts of the love object that excite him or her and will not be able to understand or perceive the whole person.

How love relations are affected by the levels of personality structure

Love requires some degree of idealization of another. How healthy the idealization depends on our personality structure. Psychoanalyst-theoretician-researcher Otto Kernberg (1985, 1995, 2002) described these three groupings of personality structure as Borderline, Neurotic, and Normal (healthy), and this formulation later became incorporated into the PDM (2006). The PDM represents the most advanced scientific formation of personality. Now let us look at these three levels of love relations according to Kernberg.

1. At the borderline level of personality organization, idealization is based on splitting. Splitting occurs when people see

themselves and others as either all good or all bad. They have difficulty accepting the complex nature of people and relate to others in terms of their needs and projections. The other person is perceived as good if they believe that person might meet their needs. The other person is perceived as bad or useless if the person does not meet their needs.

At this borderline level, a person falls in love with a part person, not a whole person. The object of desire represents erotic and dependent needs. There is a great deal of idealization without empathy for the beloved.

Borderline personalities can quickly move from intense idealization to devaluation. They fall in love with projections of their grandiose self. However, since they have problems with impulse control and aggression, the intimacy is often destroyed. This idealization is fragile.

If a person is not mature, the destructive aspects of passion kill the intimacy. Sexuality can become intense, dominated by aggression and emotional sadomasochism.

All passion requires some sadomasochism. The word "passion" originally meant "to suffer" as in "the passion of Jesus." Passionate love is primitive and aggressive. Immature individuals can be very passionate, but they end up letting their aggression or need to suffer destroy the relationship. Healthier individuals are able to keep the sadomasochism in the playful and teasing aspects of the eroticism without harming the relationship.

People with borderline personality organization unconsciously wish that ideal love and sexual gratification from the new love object would overcome their inner conflicts. Borderline personalities seek a dependent relationship and resent the person they depend on. Borderline personalities may fear imprisonment in intimacy since they project their own need to exploit and control onto the love object. They project the denied worst parts of themselves onto the partner. They also tend to act out in order to provoke the partner to react as the persecutory object. That way, they can assure themselves that they now have the power to escape from and punish the love object.

Borderline personalities fear separation from sources of security. Separations can lead to decomposition. Devaluing the object of dependency is a common defense. When faced with separation, criticism, or frustration, they project the impaired self onto the partner and go into a rage.

They tend to experience the ordinary reciprocity of human relations as exploitive and unfair. The partner must become exactly as they need him or her to be. They regard any limits as rejection.

2.   The second level is the neurotic personality organization. The idealization found with individuals having neurotic personalities is more reality-based than with the borderline level. The image of the idealized parent is transferred to the new love object to form the basis for love and conflict. Rather than problems with impulsiveness, defensiveness, and aggression that characterize the borderline level, the main problems at the neurotic level of personality organization are inhibition, anxiety, and guilt.

A person with a neurotic personality organization has the capacity for empathy and awareness of the beloved. At this level, there is remorse and concern because the conscience is well developed. However, neurosis comes with too strong a superego (conscience), so there is often sexual inhibition and guilt that compromises the intimacy.

Often, people with a neurotic personality organization and a borderline personality organization fall in love with each other. These are complementary relationships. The neurotic personality has empathy, guilt, and masochism and can put up with the exploitive, aggressive personality of the borderline. They are gratified vicariously by the borderline person's expression of sexuality and aggression without neurotic guilt. On the other hand, the borderline person often sees the neurotic personality as containing and anchoring them. This alliance is often filled with conflict and instability.

3.   Normal idealization in love is based on a stable identity and realistic awareness and appreciation of the beloved as a three-dimensional, autonomous person. The mature person has the

capacity to remain in love since the love is based on a complex perception of the other's qualities that involve abstractions such as ideals, values, and goals. The idealization is based less on overcompensations, projections, and immature transferences, and more on the reality of the person. There is erotic desire for the other with little guilt to interfere with sexuality and intimacy. The erotic desire is not primarily based on the concreteness of surface features (beauty, power) or erotic fantasy (sexual fixations), but mainly on the ever-enriching personal qualities of the beloved (humor, warmth, cleverness, and concern). These personal qualities do not become boring and help love to last.

There is an ability to identify with the other's gender. There is a high capacity for empathy, tolerance, insight, remorse, and tenderness. There is a healthy concern for the other and few problems with aggression and defensiveness.

Now let us summarize the levels of idealization in love relations.

Borderline Level: Poor relationships due to seeing the beloved as all good or all bad based on one's emotions and needs; swings from idealization to devaluation; impulsive, resents limits; looks for an ideal love that will make everything right; expecting special treatment, little empathy, there is strong defensive use of denial, projection, and provocations.

How much do you experience this level of idealization in your love relations?

None	Low		Medium		High
0	1	2	3	4	5

Neurotic Level: There is the capacity to remain in love and have empathy; idealization is mainly based on the beloved's actual good qualities, but this person often struggles with sexual inhibitions, anxiety, and guilt that affect the relationship.

How much do you experience this level of idealization in your love relations?

None	Low		Medium		High
0	1	2	3	4	5

Normal Level: Capacity to remain in love and idealize based on the beloved's actual qualities; few if any problems with commitment, impulsiveness, inhibitions, anger, and defensiveness; a high capacity for empathy, tolerance, insight, remorse, and tenderness.

How much do you experience this level of idealization in your love relations?

None	Low		Medium		High
0	1	2	3	4	5

How much does your partner (or if not in a current relationship, your last partner) experience a borderline level of idealization?

None	Low		Medium		High
0	1	2	3	4	5

How much does your partner (or if not in a current relationship, your last partner) experience a neurotic level of idealization?

None	Low		Medium		High
0	1	2	3	4	5

How much does your partner (or if not in a current relationship, your last partner) experience a normal level of idealization?

None	Low		Medium		High
0	1	2	3	4	5

9

How Defensive Styles
Affect Love Relations

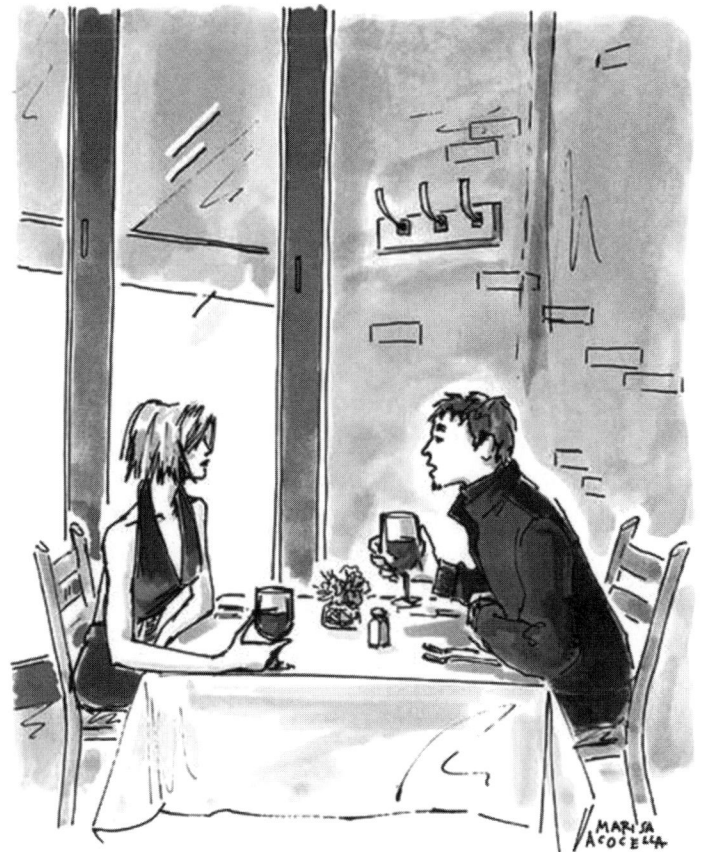

"Believe me when I tell you that I'm not that honest."

Defense mechanisms help protect a person from too much anxiety or threat to self-esteem. The healthier defenses are more conscious and constructive, such as humor or suppression, than the primitive defenses, which are unconscious and destructive, such as denial and projection. It is not being defensive when you are just defending your point of view and not distorting or denying reality. Here are some of the main defense mechanisms.

Healthy defenses found in normal (healthy) people are:

Humor—seeing the irony or absurdity in a problem (we value comedy for this reason)

Sublimation—converting aggressive or sexual tensions into socially valued behavior (such as work, hobbies, sports, or art)

Suppression—consciously pushing aside stresses and conflicts for a while

Repression—pushing out of conscious awareness both stresses and conflicts

Normal and neurotic people favor repression as a defense. Some degree of repression is necessary in life, as long as the repressed issues can at some point be retrieved and resolved. Some degree of repression helps us cope with the stresses in relationships and life. People with borderline (immature) personality organizations do not favor repression as a defense. They favor primitive defenses.

Primitive defensives are associated with individuals with borderline personality organizations.

Primitive defenses are:

Devaluation/Idealization—values others in extremes according to one's emotions and needs

Denial—refusing to acknowledge internal reality (feelings, thoughts) or external reality

Rationalization—offering rational-sounding excuses for irrational, unconscious motives

Projection—attributing one's own unacceptable feelings or motives to someone else

Projective Identification—misattributes own feelings and motives to another and then induces those feelings through provocation

Splitting—cannot experience ambiguous and ambivalent feelings or perceptions of the self or others, so the person views things in the extremes of all good or all bad

Acting out—conflicts are expressed unconsciously in behaviors rather than talked out

It is difficult to have an intimate relationship with someone who favors the primitive defenses. They will deny that they were wrong. They will not learn from their mistakes. They will project faults, provoke problems, and blame you for them.

What defenses have you used and how much?

Humor

None	Low		Medium		High
0	1	2	3	4	5

Sublimation

None	Low		Medium		High
0	1	2	3	4	5

Suppression

None	Low		Medium		High
0	1	2	3	4	5

Repression

None	Low		Medium		High
0	1	2	3	4	5

Devaluation/Idealization

None	Low		Medium		High
0	1	2	3	4	5

Denial

None	Low		Medium		High
0	1	2	3	4	5

Rationalization

None	Low		Medium		High
0	1	2	3	4	5

Projection

None	Low		Medium		High
0	1	2	3	4	5

Projective Identification

None	Low		Medium		High
0	1	2	3	4	5

Splitting

None	Low		Medium		High
0	1	2	3	4	5

Acting out

None	Low		Medium		High
0	1	2	3	4	5

If you rated them all "0" or "1," then you at least have some denial. Even normal people will use many of these defenses at some time or another! Only humor and suppression are consciously used.

Unconsciously, we favor the defenses based on our level of emotional maturity. However, at times, even a mature person will use denial. Now go back and try to think of when you have used each of these defenses. If you are stuck, your partner or friend can certainly help point out examples. (Thank them for the feedback. You must offer anyone rendering such feedback protection from resentment!)

I must be in denial for expecting people to be aware of defense mechanisms that are, by their very nature, unconscious. On the other hand, if I can catch myself using denial, then maybe some of you can also.

On Being Constructive

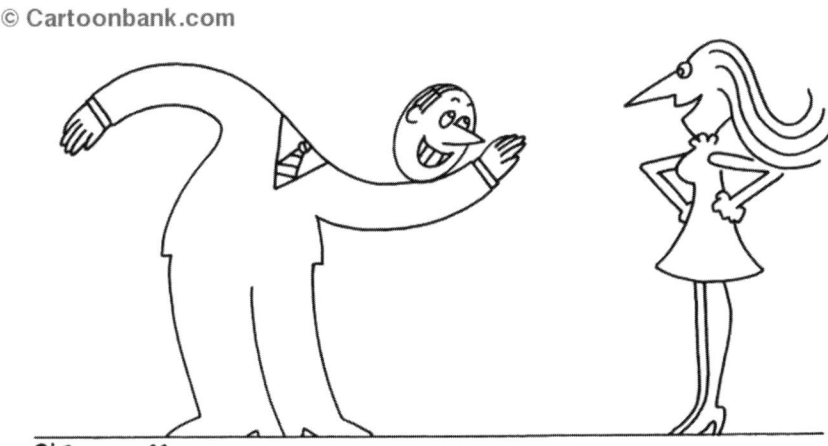

"Well, darn, Ted, I just can't stay mad at you."

The use of apology in relationships

People who favor primitive defenses have problems with a true apology. However, without an insightful, responsible, and remorseful apology, the relationship remains damaged and does not heal. Emotionally immature people see an apology as a humiliation.

However, the act of apology is an expression of maturity. It has the power to help heal wounds. The levels of apology are:

1. Refusal to apologize. This is not a sign of strength, but immaturity.
2. The use of apology to manipulate the person back into the relationship. There is no responsibility or insight. "I promise it will never happen again."
3. The apology without a sense of responsibility. "Sorry it happened."
4. The responsible but insightless apology. These people have no insight as to their motives. "I'm sorry I hurt you. Forgive me."
5. The full apology is when the person takes full responsibility, shows remorse and concern, identifies the hurtful behaviors, shows insight, and resolves to do better. "I'm sorry that I hurt you. I can see what I did. I blamed you for my mistake because I did not want to look stupid. I got defensive. I see it now. I care about you, I do not like hurting you, and I want to be a better person. I will try to do better."

How often can you give a full apology?

Never	Rarely		Sometimes		Often
0	1	2	3	4	5

How often can your partner give a full apology (or if not in a current relationship, your last partner)?

Never	Rarely		Sometimes		Often
0	1	2	3	4	5

Do you forgive and forget?

We must learn to love faulty humans. Try to forgive as much as you can after a full apology.

Forgive, but do not forget. You forget only if you do not want to learn from experience. You do not want to be enabling a repeating drama. In other words, forgiving is a virtue, but forgetting is a liability.

How forgiving are you?

Never	Rarely		Sometimes		Often
0	1	2	3	4	5

Fair fighting

All intimacies have aggression in them. The trick is to fight fair and constructively by learning to:

1. Lodge a complaint in a factual manner
2. State how you feel and what you would like
3. Express your emotions such as anger in a mature fashion
4. Stay on the topic
5. Fight to be understood, not to get your way
6. Negotiate needs, weigh evidence
7. Never be mean
8. Take time out if things escalate
9. Apologize, admit that you are wrong
10. Resolve fights quickly and get back to getting along

How fair and constructive are your fights? (If you think, "I don't fight," that is actually a sneaky way to fight).

Not Fair		Medium			Fair
0	1	2	3	4	5

All intimacies that promote personal growth have certain things in common: commitment, constructive feedback, emotional insight, concern, remorse, responsibility, and a willingness to be a better person. If these conditions are met in a love relationship, there can be personal growth and better love relations.

How well do you express the following in your intimacies?

Commitment to the relationship

None	Low		Medium		High
0	1	2	3	4	5

Constructive feedback (critical feedback that is fair and helpful)

None	Low		Medium		High
0	1	2	3	4	5

Emotional insight (understanding the internal causes of your emotional reactions based on your personality and past)

None	Low		Medium		High
0	1	2	3	4	5

Concern (about the other's welfare)

None	Low		Medium		High
0	1	2	3	4	5

Remorse (feeling sad because of the hurt you caused)

None	Low		Medium		High
0	1	2	3	4	5

Responsibility (owning both conscious and unconscious behaviors)

None	Low		Medium		High
0	1	2	3	4	5

A willingness to be a better person

None	Low		Medium		High
0	1	2	3	4	5

Review all your responses. Look at the depth, detail, relevancy, insightfulness, and honestly of your responses. Are there areas where you can give responses that are more valuable in service to your personal growth? Let these intellectual insights sink in emotionally. Feel what they mean for your life.

Congratulations for completing these exercises. No, this book did not magically transform you, but it gave you a foot in the door of change. However, these insights will soon fade and be rendered useless if you do not use them every day.

You can work hard to have personal growth to get more out of love and life. Every day life gives you choices to repeat your old patterns or to use emotional insight to disrupt them. You can choose to be insightful versus defensive, to be constructive versus destructive. It is not easy, but when you use emotional insight to disrupt an old tendency to repeat patterns, you have at that moment in time the opportunity to grow as a person. Nothing is more important in life than learning how to love well. It is all up to you.

A favor . . .

If you have any comments, corrections, or suggestions for improving this workbook, I would like to hear from you. Please send them to:

Robert M. Gordon, Ph.D., ABPP
1259 South Cedar Crest Boulevard, Suite #325
Allentown, Pennsylvania 18103-6261
Fax: 610.821.1072
mmpi@enter.net

References

Akhtar, S. (1999). *Inner Torment—Living Between Conflict and Fragmentation:* Jason Aronson Inc. New Jersey, London.

Bergmann, M. (1982). Platonic love, transference love and love in real life. *Journal of the American Psychoanalytic Association.* (30), 87–112.

Bradley, P. E., et al (1974). Parental MMPIs and certain pathological behaviors in children. *Journal of Clinical Psychology 30*, 379–382

Buss, D. M. (1994). *The evolution of desire: strategies of human mating.* New York: BasicBooks.

Cath, S. H. G., A.R.; Ross, J. M. (Ed.). (1982). *Father and Child: Developmental and Clinical Perspectives:* Little, Brown and Co. Boston.

Fisher, H. (2000). Lust, attraction, attachment: Biology and evolution of the three primary emotion systems for mating, reproduction, and parenting. *Journal of Sex Education & Therapy., 25*(1), 96–104.

Fonagy, P. G., G.; Jurist, E. L.; Target, M. (2002). *Affect Regulation, Mentalization and the Development of the Self.:* Other Press. NY.

Freud, S. (1912). The most prevalent form of degradation in erotic life. In E. Jones (Ed.), *Collected Papers In No. 10 Vol.IV:* The Hogarth Press and the Institute of Psycho-analysis. London 1950.

Freud, S. (1914/1957). On Narcissism: An Introduction. In *Standard Edition. Part XIV* (pp. 73–102): London: Hogarth Press.

Freud, S. (1937/1963). *Analysis terminable and interminable.:* New York: Collier.

Freud, S. (1910a). A Special Type of Object Made By Men. In E. Jones. (Ed.), *In Collected Papers Vol.IV* (pp. 192–202).

Gordon, R. M. (1982). Systems-object relations view of marital therapy: Revenge and reraising. In L. R. A. Wolberg, M. (Ed.), *Group and Family Therapy.:* Brunner-Mazel.

Gordon, R. M. (1998). The Medea Complex and the Parental Alienation Syndrome: When Mothers Damage Their Daughter's Ability to Love a Man. In G. H. Fenchel (Ed.), *The Mother–Daughter Relationship Echoes Through Time:* Jason Aronson Inc. Northvale, New Jersey.

Gordon, R. M. (2001). MMPI/MMPI-2 changes in long-term psychoanalytic psychotherapy. *Issues in Psychoanalytic Psychology, 23,* 59–79).

Gordon, R. M. (2005). The Doom and Gloom of Divorce Research. Comment on Wallerstein and Lewis (2004). *Psychoanalytic Psychology, 22*(3), 450–451.

Gordon, R. M. (2006d). What Is Love? A Unified Model of Love Relations. *Issues In Psychoanalytic Psychology, 28*(1), 25–33.

Gordon, R. M. (2006b and 2007). *I Love You Madly! On Passion, Personality and Personal Growth.* Charleston, S.C.: BookSurge,LLC and in 2007 IAPT Press.

Gordon, R. M. (2006d). *An Expert Look at Love, Intimacy and Personal Growth.* In. Allentown, Pa.: IAPT Press.

Harvey, J. H. (1989). People's naïve understandings of their close relationships: Attributional and personal construct perspectives. *International Journal of Personal Construct psychology., 2*(1), 37–48.

Kernberg, O. F. (1974). Barriers to falling and remaining in love. *Journal of the American Psychoanalytic Association., 22,* 486–511.

Kernberg, O. F. (1985). *Object relations theory and clinical psychoanalysis.* New York: Jason Aronson.

Kernberg, O. F. (1995). *Love relations : normality and pathology.* New Haven: Yale University Press.

Kernberg, O. F. (2002). *Borderline conditions and pathological narcissism* (Expanded ed.). Northvale, NJ: Jason Aronson.

Kuleshnyk, I. (1984). The Stockholm syndrome: Toward an understanding. *Social Action and the Law., 10*(2), 37–42.

Meston, C. a. F., P.F. (2003). Love at first fright: Partner salience moderates roller-coaster induced excitation transfer. *Archives of Sexual Behavior., 32*(6), 537–544.

Norcross, J. C. (2002). Empirically supported therapy relationships. In J. C. Norcross (Ed.), *Psychotherapy relationships that work: Therapist contributions and responsiveness to patients.* (pp. 3–16). New York, NY, US: Oxford University Press.

Panksepp, J. (1998). Affective neuroscience: The foundations of human and animal emotions. (pp. xii, 466). New York, NY, US: Oxford University Press.

Panksepp, J. (2004). Basic Affects and the Instinctual Emotional Systems of the Brain: The Primordial Sources of Sadness, Joy, and Seeking. In A. S. R. Manstead, N. Frijda & A. Fischer (Eds.), *Feelings and emotions: The Amsterdam symposium.* (pp. 174–193). New York, NY, US: Cambridge University Press.

PDM, T. F. (2006). *Psychodynamic Diagnostic Manual.* Silver Spring, MD: Alliance of Psychoanalytic Organizations.

Pines, A. (1998). *Gender and culture in romantic attraction.* Paper presented at the 24th International Congress of Applied Psychology., San Francisco, Ca.

Pines, A. M. (2001). The role of gender and culture in romantic attraction. *European Psychologist, 6*(2), 96–102.

Pines, A. M., & Zaidman, N. (2003). Gender, Culture, and Social Support: A Male-Female, Israeli Jewish-Arab Comparison. *Sex Roles, 49*(11–12), 571–586.

Pope, K. T., B.G. (1994). Therapists as patients: A national survey of psychologists' experiences, problems, and beliefs. *Professional Psychology: Research & Practice, 25*(3), 247–258.

Schore, A. N. (1994). *Affect Regulation and the Origin of the Self. The Neurobiology of Emotional Development:* Lawrence Erlbaum Assoc. New Jersey.

Stephan, W. A. B., E. and Walster, E. (1971). Sexual arousal and interpersonal perception. *Journal of Personality and Social Psychology, 20,* 93–101.

Sternberg, R. J. (1986a). A triangular theory of love. *Psychological Review, 93,* 119–135.

Walters, E. M., S.; Treboux, D.; Crowell, J. and Albersheim, L. (2000). Attachment Security in Infancy and Early Adulthood: A Twenty-Year Longitudinal Study. *Child Development, 71*(3), 684–689.

Wampold, B. E. (2001). *The great psychotherapy debate: Models, methods, and findings.:* Mahwah, NJ: Lawrence Erlbaum.

Young, A. (1997). Finding the mind's construction in the face. *Psychologist., 10*(10), 447–452.

Ziv, A. (1993). *Psychology: The Science of Understanding Human Beings.(Hebrew):* Tel Aviv: Am Oved. Cited in Ayala Malach Pines (1999) *Falling in Love: Why We Choose the Lovers We Choose.* Routledge New York.